YOUR fit PREGNANCY

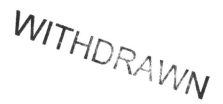

TRIMESTER -BY- TRIMESTER

YOUR fit PREGNANCY

Nutrition & Exercise
HANDBOOK

Erica Willick

STERLING
New York

STERLING
New York

An Imprint of Sterling Publishing
1166 Avenue of the Americas
New York, NY 10036

Workout photography by Carston Leishman,
Lemontree Photography Inc.
Recipe photography by Christal Sczebel,
Nutritionist in the Kitch

ISBN 978–1–4549–1693–2

Distributed in Canada by Sterling Publishing
c/o Canadian Manda Group, 664 Annette Street
Toronto, Ontario, Canada M6S 2C8
Distributed in the United Kingdom
by GMC Distribution Services
Castle Place, 166 High Street,
Lewes, East Sussex, England BN7 1XU
Distributed in Australia by Capricorn Link (Australia) Pty. Ltd.
P.O. Box 704, Windsor, NSW 2756, Australia

For information about custom editions, special sales,
and premium and corporate purchases, please contact
Sterling Special Sales at 800–805–5489
or specialsales@sterlingpublishing.com.

Manufactured in China

2 4 6 8 10 9 7 5 3 1

www.sterlingpublishing.com

Dedication

For the babies that made us stronger CURTIS & FAITH

CONTENTS

Foreword

FIRST MET ERICA WILLICK THROUGH THE INTERTWINED WEB OF SOCIAL media. I run a fitness community called Busy Mom Gets Fit, which has grown exponentially since 2011. I think Busy Mom Gets Fit has been successful because of the message of strength over skinny, hard work over a quick fix, and empowering yourself all while being a busy mom. I am a mother of four boys, and my community has become part of my journey as we continue to seek strength and balance despite our crazy lives.

I recognized that we women are powerful when we join forces and I personally desired the support of like-minded social media women—other busy moms who are building up other moms (or moms-to-be)—so I started the Mom Power Team. I received Erica's application in 2012 right after she won the North American professional level fitness show for bikini and started appearing in Oxygen magazine. But I saw that her mission, way more important than titles and magazine pages, was similar to my own. Erica became part of the founding twenty members of the influential Mom Power Team, which has a reach of close to one million women.

Through our interactions, Erica and I shared some crazy ideas—like changing the world. The only difference between Erica and me and most people was that we took each other seriously! After a few half-joking and then some serious international conversations, and before meeting in person, Erica and I decided to take the leap to create a magazine. A brand. A culture that we craved. We partnered up and created *Gorgo Women's Fitness Magazine*. We were fed up with what we saw being glamorized as women's fitness—we were craving more. We wanted more real information written for smart women, more real workouts, and more real nutrition advice. The name Gorgo sometimes strikes people as odd, but once they know the meaning behind it, women around the world call themselves #GorgoGirls. We named our magazine after the ancient Greek Spartan queen Gorgo. The Spartan culture believed that strong women produce strong heirs. As a result, Spartans actually encouraged their girls to train alongside boys.

As a pregnant woman you'd be interested to know that historians believe that Spartan women had more live births than their ancient Greek counterparts and infant mortality was lower because the women were healthier when they conceived and ate better during pregnancy. Looks like not much has changed in more than 2,000 years.

Erica is one of the smartest people I know. I've watched her balance a busy life as a working mom and still thrive in her health and fitness. She's a forward and deep thinker, and her heart is in helping other women. She's brought a lot of women along with her through her coaching and Sisters in Shape community—women just like you who are living real lives and trying to do their best with their health. She is an expert researcher and is in constant pursuit of the best—the best methods for exercise, the best systems for nutrition, the best solutions for real life.

One of the key aspects of Erica's personality is her encouragement of other women. She's deeply committed to her purpose of empowering women in their health and fitness, so they in turn can thrive and fulfill their purpose in life, as mothers, as wives, as career women.

I'm certain under Erica's no-compromise pursuit of the best, *Your Fit Pregnancy* contains the best information available to pregnant women on all aspects of health and fitness. Not only that, but that these are doable solutions that can actually work in your real life.

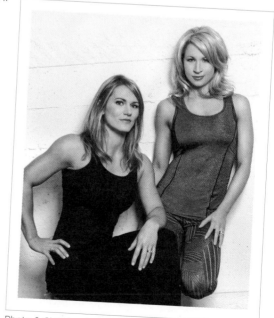

Photo & Clothing: MPG Sport

VALERIE SOLOMON
February 2015
Busymomgetsfit.com

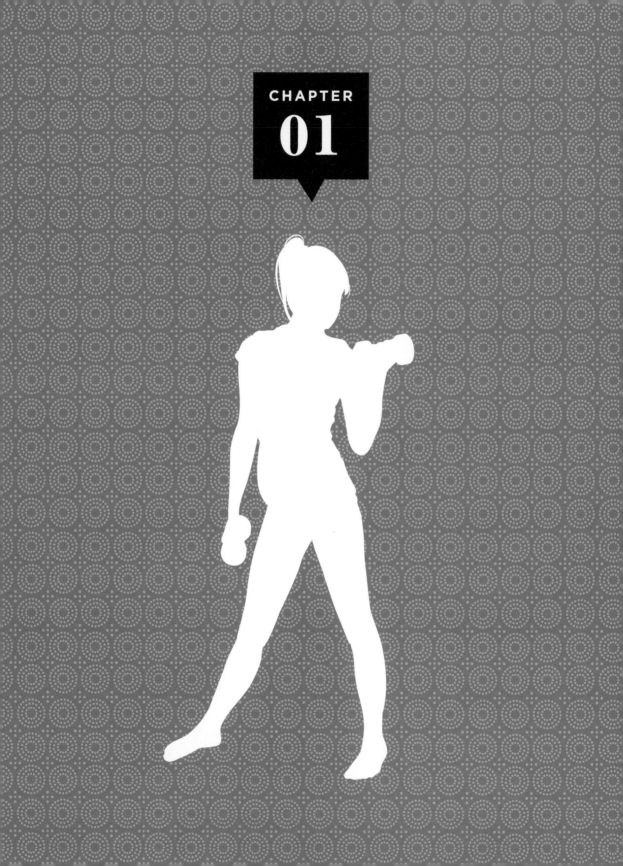

CHAPTER

01

YOUR FIT AND HEALTHY PREGNANCY

→ Ready to start one of the most amazing (and challenging) journeys of your life? Let's peel back the layers of being fit with baby-on-board.

This is not another guilt trip. This book is not going to begin with a laundry list of the benefits to mommy and baby of healthy eating and exercise. As women we are already inundated with countless "shoulds" that stack up. Piles of dishes, work assignments, kids' projects, gym sneakers, and that fancy unused food processor all remind us of all the things we "should" be doing to be a great wife/mom/employee/daughter/friend. Oh yes, and there's the pressure to look great while doing all of that.

And a pregnant woman? Well, she is blessed with carrying a precious new life, so she also has the honor of being blessed with a "should" list that is twice as long and full of conflicting advice, and no magic fairy to come and take away her existing "should" list. Oh yes, you "should" look glowing while doing all of that.

Sound like a rant? I say it sounds like reality.

Empowering Information + Love + Practical Solutions

The news of baby number 2 came to me at a time when I felt in control of my body and life. I would be considered "very fit" by most standards—I even learned about my second pregnancy just a couple of weeks after winning a North American professional level natural fitness competition (bikini division, which means I looked cute and fit on stage in a bikini and heels!). Don't roll your eyes just yet! There's more depth to this woman than a sparkly bikini. In reality I worked full-time as a corporate finance professional and had an energetic four-year-old son and a very supportive husband. Fitness was my "hobby." As part of my "hobby" I cofounded and run a growing women's fitness magazine, as well as a successful online health and fitness coaching business. Both of these side fitness projects were founded on the principles of empowering women in their health and helping them discover their strength. Yes, I was "busy," but I had a deep love and sense of purpose for what I was bringing to the world of women's health and fitness.

Yet within one week of the blessed pregnancy news, I was completely humbled by pregnancy-related sickness, exhaustion, bloating, and food aversions that lasted 24/7. Thirteen weeks passed before I was granted reprieve. Just as I entered my second trimester, I felt good enough to crawl off my then habitual spot on the couch, and I wondered "What now?!"

I knew the power of healthy living, since it had transformed my life three and a half years earlier following the birth of my first child. From firsthand experience, plenty of research, and working with hundreds of other busy modern women, I knew the physical and mental benefits of healthy living. But did the same methods of nutrition and exercise apply now that I was pregnant? I had a precious life growing inside me, so was it okay for me to keep doing what I did before pregnancy? I certainly didn't feel the same as before—my body was rebelling, I was tired, and healthy foods and I were not currently friends. Yet a key lesson in adopting a healthy lifestyle kept calling to me: never (ever) give up. So at 14 weeks pregnant, I went back to square one.

I sought out the most-up-to-date, quality research on pregnancy, nutrition, and exercise; I spoke with doctors, physiotherapists, and other experts about my questions. I also learned from other women who had lived through the ups and downs of staying fit while pregnant. Unfortunately, I quickly found that much of the available information on the topics that I craved to know about was either fragmented into silos or barely scratched the surface on how to actually apply nutrition,

exercise, and lifestyle advice to a busy (real) life throughout your entire pregnancy. So I rolled up my sleeves, pulled it all together into usable programs, tested it, tweaked it, and then altered it over and over again as my body kept changing.

I've packaged my insights into *Your Fit Pregnancy* so I can share with you in detail the whys and how-tos of being healthy and fit during pregnancy. I will be here throughout your pregnancy journey and beyond to gently encourage you in the way a good friend or sister would. She would remind you not to be too hard on yourself, that no one is perfect, and that you and baby are worth never (ever) giving up on.

One of the first people I shared my pregnancy news with was my sister Andrea. I told her I had news, and she responded, "I have news, too." We were shocked to find out we were both expecting—on the same day! Andrea and I were both heavily interested in healthy eating and fitness; Andrea worked as a yoga and group fitness instructor along with raising her three-year-old daughter. We both led very different day-to-day lives and had very different experiences during our pregnancies (neither "easy" or "glowing"), yet we both committed to being healthy and fit throughout our pregnancies.

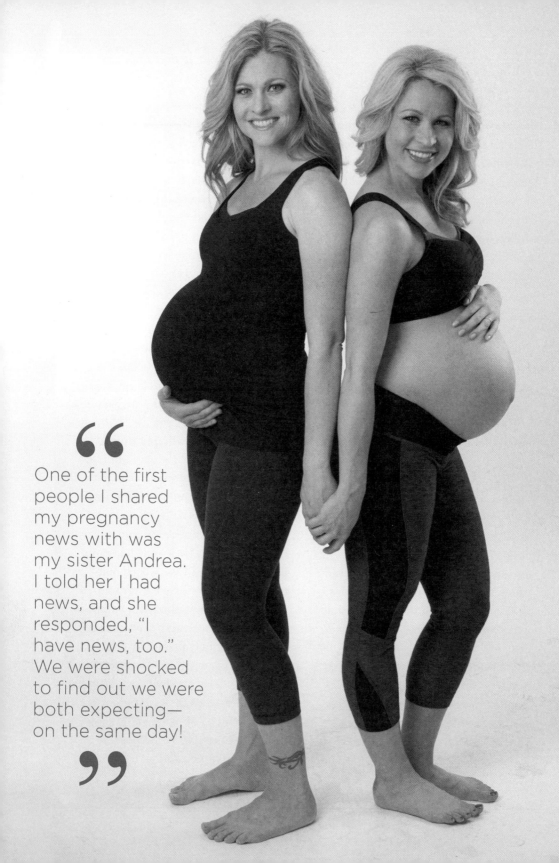

> One of the first people I shared my pregnancy news with was my sister Andrea. I told her I had news, and she responded, "I have news, too." We were shocked to find out we were both expecting—on the same day!

Having a sisterly voice to help navigate through the confusing information and empathize with during inevitable downs made a world of difference to sticking to our commitment.

My dream is that this book becomes your sisterly voice and serves as a useful tool throughout one of the most incredible journeys of your life. Whether you are brand new to healthy living and exercise or an experienced gym warrior, these principles and programs were made to help you navigate through your pregnancy journey healthier and even fitter. A woman needs empowering information, love, and practical solutions to do what is best for herself and baby.

Your Fit Pregnancy Exercise

What the heck is a "fit" pregnant woman? Fit is a funny word, as I've seen it used to describe a wide range of women. An Olympic athlete is obviously "fit," and yet the same word could be used to describe your fit friend Suzie who jogs three miles every morning. The woman pumping a 40-pound barbell in your gym's weight room would be "fit," right? Yet, so would your yoga instructor who wraps her legs around her shoulders in a double-up-down-bird-tree-dog pose. So "fit" clearly isn't reserved to just one activity, nor is it a label that describes just one level.

Maybe we can pinpoint what "fit" looks like then? Hmmm . . . an Olympic swimmer has a very different look than an Olympic gymnast. A world-class tennis player looks very different from a CrossFit athlete. Even within the same activity, especially in general fitness, many women look completely different and still rock at "being fit."

One of my favorite representations of what "fit looks like" was taken at one of our recent Gorgo magazine photo shoots. We lined up thirteen very fit women (and one baby) to show what "fit" really looks like. The result? Fit didn't look like one thing. The cool thing about fit is that fit looks beautiful in so many different shapes and sizes.

I'll tell you what fit is not—fit is not leanness. Leanness is leanness. Lean is often used to describe a lower ratio of body fat to muscle. If a woman has some muscle developed and if she has a lower body fat ratio, you can see the outlines and shape of the muscle she has developed. You could have a lot of muscle and be very fit, but if it's covered with a layer of fat, you will not look as toned as a woman with lower body fat who has the same amount of muscle. Without developed muscles, a woman with low body fat is often described as looking "skinny."

Why am I talking about "leanness" and "skinny" in a pregnancy book? In our image-driven culture, understanding this concept is important for resetting your expectations about what "fit" really is compared to what too many think fit looks like (i.e., "lean"). Can you imagine a pregnant woman telling her friends her goal was to be "lean" during her pregnancy instead of explaining that her goal was to stay

fit? That's nuts—not to mention potentially unhealthy for baby. Yet, many women aren't aware that the "fit look" they see in our image-driven culture is actually leanness, not fitness.

I received a message from a pregnant woman asking how she could avoid losing all the muscle definition she worked hard to develop pre-baby. Aside from continuing her strength training, I coached her to understand that adding body fat is important for baby's health during pregnancy. Additional fat is needed

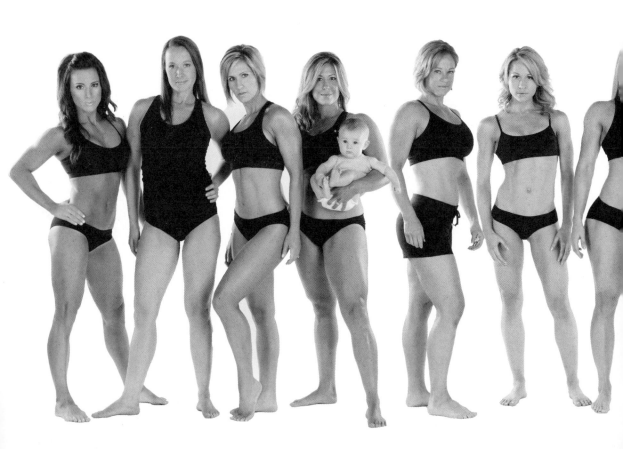

during pregnancy as an energy reserve for baby in case of hard times such as an illness, and it also functions as stored energy for milk production postpartum. That additional body fat, not to mention the typical water retention experienced in most pregnancies, would likely hide those beautiful biceps she worked hard to develop, because seeing definition requires a certain level of leanness. Notice how I said "hide," not lose. For most of my fitness clients, 5–10 pounds is often the difference between seeing definition

or not. They can be very fit but lack the leanness (low body fat/muscle ratio) to look fit by our society's current standards.

It is a well-accepted guideline that a healthy weight gain during pregnancy is 25–35 pounds (11.5–16 kilograms) for women at a normal pre-pregnancy weight for their height. For overweight and obese woman, less weight should be gained, typically no more than 20 pounds (9 kilograms). That weight gain is not all body fat. Of the 25–35 pounds you're actually likely to gain

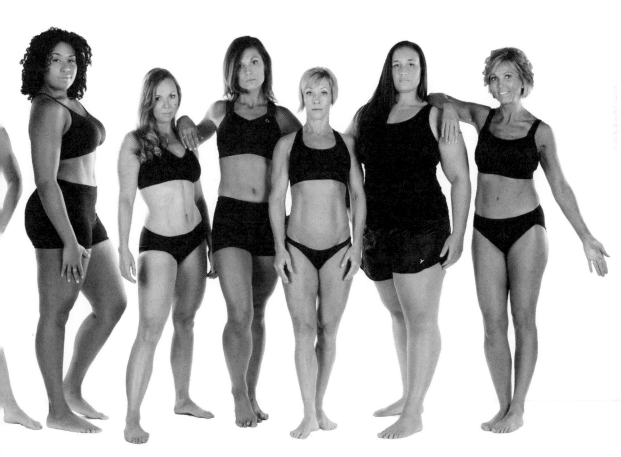

only 7–10 pounds of that as fat; the rest of the weight gain is from your enlarged uterus, placenta, breast tissue, and amniotic fluid. But regardless, the additional body fat and fluid make it difficult if not impossible to keep the lean look many women mistake as "fit."

Hopefully by now I've convinced you that fit comes in all shapes, sizes, levels, and activities, that lean does not equal "fit," and that lean should not be a goal for your pregnancy. So what the heck is a "fit pregnant woman"?! She is one who is active in the ways her body can move. She consistently works on her strength and heart so that baby has a healthier start to life. She isn't perfect or even hard-core. To show you this firsthand, I've included a "Preggo Pal Profile" in each chapter so you can see examples of other woman who were fit during their pregnancy. The spectrum of their looks and fitness demonstrates how being a "fit pregnant woman" isn't about being like me—it is about being the best you.

You Are a Natural Bodybuilder

Don't freak. We are not talking about getting all muscled-up like Arnold Schwarzenegger. But did you know that you are currently the world's most natural bodybuilder? You are literally building a body inside of you! From toes that wiggle, a heart that beats, and eyes that blink, you are constructing another human from the inside out. Any traditional bodybuilder will tell you that it's their nutrition and exercise choices that shaped their end result. And while all the recent studies will point to the benefits of exercising and eating well during pregnancy, this knowledge was woven into the ancient Greek Spartan culture more than 2,000 years ago.

The Spartans believed that strong women produced strong heirs and encouraged their girls to train with the boys. That was 2,000 years ago, and yet today we too often struggle with our girls and women being encouraged to be active and strong. As a nod to this ancient culture, my business partner and I named our women's fitness magazine Gorgo after a Spartan queen.

Historians believe that Spartans had more live births than their counterparts from other city-states and that infant mortality was lower because Spartan women were healthier when they conceived and ate better during pregnancy. Fast-forward more than 2,000 years, and

Mommy & Baby Benefits of Exercising During Pregnancy

- Labor and delivery may be easier
- Boosts baby's brain maturity
- Reduces mommy's blood pressure
- Lowers gestational diabetes risk by as much as 41 percent
- Increased energy
- Better sleep
- Baby less likely to become an overweight child
- Less likely to need forceps delivery, C-section, or other intervention
- Less prone to morning sickness
- May boost child's athletic potential
- Develops a healthier heart for baby that lasts into childhood

science continues to confirm what the ancient Spartans already knew.

Somewhere in those 2,000 years, the Spartans' cultural knowledge was overtaken by the image of women being "delicate," even helpless, especially during pregnancy. I found adopting an "I am a bodybuilder" mantra during my pregnancy empowering, as it provided me strength and reassurance about making informed choices about my nutrition and exercise, despite many cultural objections to my picking up the weights and staying active while I built one of the most important bodies of my life (my new baby's body and the one I would bring her into the world with—mine!).

Fitness Basics: Baby on Board

IF IT DOESN'T FEEL RIGHT, DON'T DO IT! I started my pregnancy journey following the common and well-accepted advice of "if you were doing that exercise before pregnancy, then you're okay to continue it during your pregnancy." I quickly learned that this advice was not intended to be followed literally, as some moves and routines that were standard before didn't feel right even just five weeks into the pregnancy. I would attempt an exercise routine that was straightforward for me to complete pre-pregnancy and I found myself breathless before I was halfway through. My gut told me to stop even though the intensity and exercise move had been relatively easy for me pre-pregnancy. While I knew instinctively I was making the right choice by stopping what didn't feel right, I felt like a failure because that common advice suggested that I should have been able to "keep it up," at least at the beginning. However, as I worked through accepting my new and ever-changing abilities, I learned that the better advice is to be 100 percent present during your workouts so you that you can listen to and respect what your body is telling you.

STRENGTH TRAIN: Strength training can be done with dumbbells, resistance bands, machines, and even your own body weight. Keep in mind that I'm not talking about monster box jumps wearing a weighted vest. *Your Fit Pregnancy*'s strength training exercises are low impact while still providing cardiovascular benefits. Strength training is key to staying injury-free, especially when a little weighted action works the tendons and ligaments that support the muscles that are in major demand when carrying around a growing baby bump. You also strengthen your bones with strength training; this is especially important for pregnant women as your growing baby is pulling calcium from your bones. Finally, preserving (even building) muscle throughout your pregnancy can be your secret weapon to regaining your shape post-baby.

BUILD UP BABY'S CARDIO: Any activity that gets your heart rate up is cardiovascular exercise. Think briskly walking, swimming, or hitting the elliptical at the gym. My separate cardio time was most frequently accomplished with family walks after dinner. A baby's heart rate rises in unison with her mother's, as if the child were also working out. Scientists believe that, as a result, babies born to active mothers tend to have better cardiovascular systems. Some studies suggest that these cardiovascular benefits last well into early childhood.

GET YOUR ZEN ON: Prenatal yoga and stretching have soared in popularity recently, and for good reason. I found no better solution to dealing with tension in my low back, hips, chest, and upper back than a gentle prenatal stretch session. As baby grows, more stress is put on these specific muscle groups. Even a short 15-minute stretching and deep breathing session can do the trick to calm your nervous system, aid with digestion, and improve sleep as well as your immune system.

AIM FOR 30 MINUTES OF ACTIVITY EVERY DAY: Every day?! Yes, every day. I was surprised at this recommendation, as it is common to see "rest days" in exercise programs. Cultural norms for pregnant women would be surprised with this advice, as I couldn't keep count of the number of times I was asked by friends and acquaintances, "Are you still exercising?" But as the American Congress of Obstetricians and Gynecologists (AOCG), which makes this recommendation, points out, "Pregnant women should be encouraged to engage in regular, moderate-intensity physical activity to continue to derive the same health benefits during their pregnancies as they did prior to pregnancy." Being active doesn't mean you are working out every day or even doing activity in a continuous 30-minute session. It means you're moving your bum and that bump daily. Even two 15-minute walks can do the trick.

CONSISTENCY TRUMPS PERFECTION: So today you feel like you got hit by a truck or you're gonna toss your cookies. And you feel that way tomorrow, and the next day. The couch and your bed are the only two places that seem to be worth movement. Don't "should" yourself into feeling worse—like Rome, your baby isn't built in one day. For two miserable months during the first trimester, I was more inconsistent than consistent. So I started following the *Your Fit Pregnancy* principles when I could and reaped all of the benefits discussed in this program, because consistency always trumps the ideal of perfection.

CHANGE WHEN YOUR BODY CHANGES: Just when you think you're catching a groove, your body moves on to the next baby-building phase, and what was working before doesn't feel right anymore. I found this especially demotivating early in pregnancy, as your new pregnancy hormones are showing you just how little control you have over your body. Perhaps I'm stubborn, but it took me several weeks to accept that my body had changed, then it finally clicked for me and I accepted that my body was changing with or without my consent. Acceptance of these continuous changes empowered me to move forward and have a healthy and fit pregnancy. As your pregnancy progresses, the size of your stomach makes exercise selections tricky, and your need for stability during activity increases. *Your Fit Pregnancy* is designed with your trimester-specific body in mind, but if your body changes faster (or slower), accept it and move on to a different program that may work better for your ever-changing body.

Your Fit Pregnancy Nutrition

You'll hear people say, "You're eating for two!" and actually encourage you to load up on your portions or indulge in treats. Yes, you are literally eating for two, as what you put into your mouth must nourish both you and baby. But don't interpret that common saying as an invitation to eat excessive portions and treats. We all know our baby's nutrition comes from us, but did you know that your growing fetus can't digest its own food?

This is a fascinating pregnancy fact you'll want to tell all of your pregnant friends and share at the next dinner party you attend: Did you know that your baby in utero cannot physically turn food into nutrients on her own because she lacks the bacteria in her stomach required to digest food? She lacks even the good kind of bacteria, because your placenta screens out all bacteria (good and bad) so that the fetus can survive in utero. This means that your baby is born without the good

bacteria needed to digest food on her own. So how does your baby get that first dose of bacteria? If you deliver vaginally, then your baby gets her first beneficial bacteria directly from your vagina (aka vagina-faced). Don't say "yuck," say "wow!" Your vagina is full of lactic acid bacteria, the good kind of bacteria that can metabolize milk. When she exits the birth canal, your baby's face and mouth are coated with this good bacteria so that she can start digesting on her own. Before she was vagina-faced, it wasn't possible for her to digest food into nutrients, so instead you digested your food and then pipelined the nutrients you ate into her through the umbilical cord. Kinda cool, right?

If your baby is born by C-section, her first digestive bacteria come from the people who hold her or the environment she's born into. Unfortunately, not all bacteria are created equal. Initial studies are showing that the bacteria from your vagina is better for baby and can positively impact her short- and long-term health. The increase in delivery by C-section in recent years has been linked to the rise in allergies, asthma, type 1 diabetes, and childhood obesity. Researchers believe this is from the initial better "gut health" provided to vaginally delivered babies.

Dr. Maria Gloria Dominguez-Bello at New York University is studying this area in depth, even testing procedures with healthy pregnant woman who need to have a C-section. Babies' faces are being smeared with gauze inserted into mom's vaginal canal in an attempt to replicate the bacteria baby would have encountered if she were born vaginally. Are you starting to get the picture of how powerful your body is right now?

So now that I've got your attention (the vagina story usually gets moms-to-be perked up and ready to listen about nutrition), can you see how important your nutrition is before baby can digest her own food? The food you put into your mouth is digested in your stomach because baby cannot digest it herself.

In digestion you break down your food into glucose, fats, and proteins. The nutrients are then absorbed into your blood and passed from you to baby through the placenta. Your placenta is a very efficient filter that rejects harmful elements, such as the bacteria that your baby can't handle yet. Smaller elements can pass through the barrier, such as oxygen, glucose, fats, proteins, vitamins, and minerals. After they enter the bloodstream, these elements are passed on to your baby through the umbilical cord.

Now imagine taking a French fry or a sugary treat and putting it into your mouth. Your stomach breaks down your fries and the sugary treat into their nutrient form and passes that on to your baby. In the case of the fries and the sugary treat it's primarily glucose and saturated fats. There are few or no proteins, vitamins, or minerals being shared with baby, and I agree that in this way you are eating for two. Now turn around how you interpret that typical phrase and eat what you would want your baby to eat—she's counting on you to give her a healthy birth weight, improve her brain development, reduce the risk of certain birth defects, and make it more likely that she'll be a healthy child and even adult. All that comes from the power of your nutrition.

Food Fundamentals and Preggo Power Foods

If you don't currently know much about nutrition, now is the best time to become an amateur nutritionist! Unfortunately, our culture's diet mentality and quick-fix fad programs have screwed up most of our understanding of nutrition. Add the food marketers into the mix—you know, those guys whose single goal is to get you to buy their product—and it's no wonder that we don't know what to eat anymore. Too many clients come to me completely overwhelmed and say, "Just tell me what to eat!" They are so confused and turned around by our current cultural norms with food that they need help with basic nutrition skills. One look at our obesity rate and lifestyle-related diseases and it is obvious that common knowledge about nutrition is no longer very common.

Dictating "eat-this-not-that" is neither my style nor the approach I've used to successfully empower my clients and fitness community. While I've included sample meal plans in each trimester and loads of recipes in this book, this was done to give you examples of how to put the fundamentals and Preggo Power Foods into a manageable and practical program for us busy ladies. But it's important that we don't start and stop there. While many clients seek me out looking for a program, I insist they learn in the process so that they don't need me in the future. My goal with clients is to work myself out of the job! It's no different here in *Your Fit Pregnancy* as I share with you the key knowledge you need to empower yourself to take control of your health and your baby's health.

The cool thing about pregnancy nutrition is that the fundamentals of eating with baby on board are mostly the same as those before and after baby. Sure, there are a few tweaks as science has shown us some special nutrients and vitamins that are powerhouses for baby building. But by learning the fundamentals, you're well on your way to being healthy for life!

Here are the three fundamentals that we will get to know intimately in other chapters and that are woven into every meal plan and recipe in *Your Fit Pregnancy*:

1. **Macronutrients (carbohydrates, proteins, and fats)**

2. **Water**

3. **Micronutrients (vitamins and minerals)**

I bet you already know at least one thing on that list (come on, you know water!), so woo-hoo, you're a third of the way there! And I know you can handle two new concepts on nutrition, because if you can take the time to figure out how to use one of those diaper gadgets you'll inevitably get as a baby gift, then something as important and powerful for your baby as nutrition won't take a backseat.

PREGGO PAL PROFILE   Meaghan Terzis

" I Committed to Just 20 Minutes a Day "

BEING A MOM is the most important job in the world. Having two amazing kids is everything to me, and I love being a full-time mom. My other passion is fitness; however, being a mom *and* being fit collided during my second pregnancy, as I was sick 24/7 for the entire nine months. I'm not talking queasy; I'm talking about around-the-clock debilitating nausea.

Medication helped subdue the sickness to make the nausea manageable. So "being fit" in the ways I used to, in the ways that I loved, was not possible. So I fell into a rut. A big one. Being active is a joy and I felt robbed of that until I shifted my mentality about what I could do in fitness.

I have a treadmill at home, and I told myself "Meaghan, just 20 minutes a day. No matter what, you can do just 20 minutes a day on that." And so I did. For my entire pregnancy, I did what I could and moved 20 minutes a day. Some days I made it 30 minutes, and on the really good days I did 40 minutes! No records were set, but I did it—I moved. I moved for me and I moved for my baby.

My son Jack was born, a healthy 6 pounds, 9 ounces, and as time went by I slowly I got back into fitness. Looking back I'm grateful I did my best and didn't get hung up about being "super-fit-preggo-mom"! I was better for it, and so was Jack. If I let it all go, I think I would have had a more difficult labor and my mentality would have been worse. It made me feel better that I did what I could.

> You can connect with Meaghan, a lovable and genuinely kind woman (and international fitness cover model!) on her public social media profiles, @meaghanterzis.

DATE: _____

DEAR BABY: _____

THE BEGINNING OF OUR JOURNEY

I want to be healthy & strong in my pregnancy because: _____

_____

_____

_____

_____

_____

_____

My goals for OUR health & wellness during pregnancy: _____

_____

_____

_____

_____

_____

_____

XOXO, Mommy

Notes: _____

_____

_____

_____

_____

_____

_____

_____

_____

_____

_____

_____

_____

_____

_____

_____

_____

_____

_____

_____

_____

_____

_____

_____

_____

_____

Notes: _____

_____

_____

_____

_____

_____

_____

_____

_____

_____

_____

_____

_____

_____

_____

_____

_____

_____

_____

_____

_____

_____

_____

_____

_____

Notes: _____

_____

_____

_____

_____

_____

_____

_____

_____

_____

_____

_____

_____

_____

_____

_____

_____

_____

_____

_____

_____

_____

_____

_____

_____

_____

_____

_____

_____

_____

CHAPTER
02

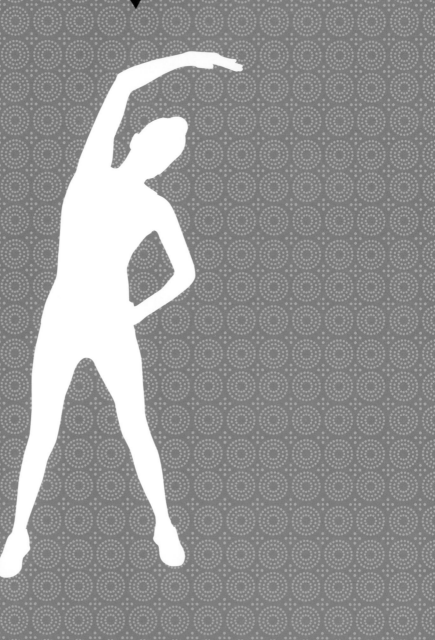

YOUR FIT FIRST TRIMESTER

→ You need building blocks to lay a strong foundation. This first trimester gives you a fresh view on your health as you create the best start for both you and baby!

Your Fit First Trimester Exercise

The most important question for a mommy-to-be is "Is it safe?" Safe for baby *and* safe for mommy. Yet this question has to be one of the most frustrating ones for a pregnant woman to get an answer to. On one hand, we're told we should exercise by the authoritative organization in prenatal health, the American College of Obstetricians and Gynecologists (ACOG). But on the other hand, it's unclear to most of us what exactly is actually safe to do and what we should avoid.

Applying our common sense, we know that there cannot be a one-size-fits-all approach—of course there are higher-risk pregnancies and individual medical situations that need to be taken into consideration. But if you're like me, you're looking for clearer general guidelines than "you should exercise" that are supported by up-to-date research and put into a framework so that you can make an educated decision with your doctor.

Let's take a look at the guidance first and create a framework for you to discuss the issue with your doctor. The AOCG says, "In the absence of either medical or obstetric complications, thirty minutes or more of moderate exercise a day on most, if not all, days of the week is recommended to pregnant women."

Okay, cool, I get that I'm supposed to be exercising for 30 minutes most days, if not every day, but that guidance is pretty vague. What exactly can and can't I do? So I look for more. Reading through the full AOCG's committee opinion is a bit tedious, but I'm committed to do what's best for baby and me, so I extract the key points from this academic written opinion. Of course it's full of caveats (remember, you're unique and you ask your doctor if there's anything special you should be taking into consideration). This is what I extract: no scuba diving (uhhh . . . duh) and avoid playing contact sports that could result in "abdominal trauma" (uhhh . . . double duh). I'm left hanging on key questions that I think apply to the average woman and how she stays active: Is running safe? Is working out safe? Are there exercises I should avoid in my general fitness other than scuba diving, contact sports, or falling over? Are there certain exercises that would be really beneficial to me and baby?

I chat with my doctor about working out during my pregnancy, and he gives me the general "If you were doing it before, you can continue. But take it easy." Hmmm . . . not a lot to work with there, and my gut is telling me there's more to it than that. Okay, time to dig in! I read the most recent research papers, speak with experts in the field of prenatal health and exercise, and reach out to other women who "stayed fit" during their pregnancy (my Preggo Pals, who are featured throughout this book). I then speak to my doctor again, and after the green light is given, I test all of this on my own pregnant body. Yes, I'm that person who will read a research paper and contact the person who wrote it to ask more questions until I have an actionable solution. The cool thing is how willing people are to share their knowledge when they are passionate about a topic. As proof, you are holding this book filled with knowledge and tips that I just had to share with my pregnant friends, clients, and those who like me sought more when all they got at first were vague directions or opinions from their mom/aunt/coworker.

A Framework for Safe and Effective Exercise

You may be surprised what you need to consider before lunging into a fitness program while you are pregnant. You're working with a whole different body with baby on board, so don't skip over these four steps as well as the suggestions on how exactly to check in with your doctor about your program.

Step 1: What Level Are You Now?

Your Fit Pregnancy provides programs and exercises for varying starting levels: beginner, intermediate, and advanced. How would you classify yourself based on these guidelines?

A) BEGINNER: You have not been active regularly, at least three times a week, in the past two months, and you are a complete newbie when it comes to strength training. You may like to walk, jog, or play a sport a couple times a week, or you may be mostly inactive.

B) INTERMEDIATE: You have been active at least three times a week in the past two months and you have some experience with strength training so that you can perform basic strength movements with good form. You can perform 30 minutes of moderate activity without any real challenge.

C) ADVANCED: You have worked out regularly (four to five times a week) in the past two months and are familiar with strength training such that you can identify and use proper form with all exercises. You can perform 30–60 minutes of moderate activity without any real challenge.

Step 2: Include Priority Preggo Exercises First

There are two priorities in your fitness during your pregnancy: moderate cardio and exercising your middle parts. Anything additional is icing on *Your Fit Pregnancy* cake!

Your middle parts are your abs, pelvic floor, glutes, hips, and low back. There is an entire chapter on this area (chapter 3: Core Confidence and Pelvic Floor Power) because it is so important and I want to ensure you are choosing safe and effective options.

If you can't do much exercise due to morning sickness, fatigue, or the many other pregnancy-related physical challenges, these two priority items should become your focus. Don't get overwhelmed or down on yourself if these are the *only* two things you can do during your entire pregnancy. If you include these two items during your pregnancy, then you had a fit pregnancy!

Step 3: Choose Your Moderate Cardio Activity

Heart health and cardiovascular health are important for you and baby! As your heart rate increases, so does your baby's heart rate. This means that when you exercise, your baby is getting in her training, too. At first this piece of research concerned me, as I pictured my baby's tiny heart racing as I exercised; however, numerous studies have found that exercising your baby's heart before she is born improves her little cardiovascular system for years after birth. I wanted my daughter to be able to race around the soccer field with a strong heart, so I gave her little heart a gentle workout by raising mine at a moderate level most days.

HEART RATE UP, BUT HOW HIGH?

Older prenatal guidance actually prescribed a maximum heart rate, but that guidance has been updated to a more general direction: ensure that you could carry on a normal conversation during your exercise activity. See pages 76–77 for more information on exercise intensity and power of pace.

THE IMPACT OF HIGH IMPACT

While most cardio activities are safe for baby during pregnancy, the higher-impact options (like running) may not be the safest choice for you. You may say "Ahhh! I *need* to run!" Don't freak out yet—I'm not going to tell you not to run, as I personally jogged a bit and know many women who ran throughout their entire pregnancies. However, I do want to give you some information so you can decide how much jogging you want to include in your pregnancy so you don't have a "Why didn't someone tell me that?" moment later on.

RUNNING AND RELAXIN
Relaxin: I'm talking about the pregnancy hormone, not chillin' out. The main job of the hormone relaxin is to help your pelvis adjust and widen for baby to descend through your birth canal. It also has the effect of relaxing *all* of your joints, muscles, tendons, and tissues in your pregnant body. This means that relaxin also affects your pelvic floor, because it's a muscle, too! As your baby and uterus grow, you add weight onto your relaxed pelvic floor muscles. How good of an idea is it to be pounding or bouncing that extra weight onto a relaxed pelvic floor muscle? We don't want to increase your chances of bladder leaks or other serious pelvic floor dysfunctions, so if you do high-impact exercise during your pregnancy

(and running is high impact), you are increasing your chances of pelvic floor dysfunction.

Does this mean you don't run during pregnancy? You'll have to make that decision for yourself, but at least you have the information to know why you may want to switch to a lower-impact cardio activity or pull back on your five-days-a-week jogging routine. Perhaps you'll choose to do an occasional jog to help you de-stress or maybe you'll continue to run five days a week. Either is okay and safe for baby, but keep in mind that there could be a negative impact for you. An empowered pregnancy is one where you have the information to make an educated decision for yourself.

While I normally run regularly, because of the information about pelvic floor muscles being compromised because of hormone changes, I decided to switch to walking outside or walking on a treadmill during my pregnancy. I liked the elliptical machine, too, as it was gentle on my joints. My top cardio choice was paced strength training, and I've included my routines here for you in *Your Fit Pregnancy* for each trimester. In my third trimester, when my joints were feeling a lot of pressure with all the extra weight I was carrying around, I did some "swimming" (aka floating like a whale supported by a pool noodle, kicking my feet a bit). These were my go-to moderate cardio options because they had low impact on my changing pregnant body and got my heart rate up.

Step 4: Strengthen Your Baby Body!

For labor and beyond, you want to build a body that is strong from head to toe. Remember, right now you are the world's most natural bodybuilder. Soon you'll be hauling around a growing newborn and bending over to pick up a loaded car seat, and soon enough that same body will be chasing around a toddler. We want to build a body that can stand up to the demands of motherhood and life! As an added benefit, muscle development will help you get that toned look many women want postpartum quicker.

All women, including pregnant women, can benefit from strength training, particularly as it relates to the improvements to your bone density. Weight-bearing exercises build more than just stronger muscles—they build stronger bones, too! This doesn't mean you need to sling around heavy weights during your pregnancy to get the benefits of strength training. A beginner can use her own body weight, as indicated in the trimester-by-trimester strength programs in this book, and an advanced exerciser can modify her favorite moves to continue being a muscle mama. A few key tips about your choice of strength training exercises:

1. Keep in mind that you have priority areas that need to be strengthened, so when you're short on time or energy those come first! Refer to step 2 of this framework.

2. After the first trimester, avoid performing exercises lying flat on your back, as that could reduce blood flow to your baby. Don't freak out if you're on your back for a couple of minutes. It's repeated and lengthy periods we're concerned about as a precaution. I have given you more than one hundred exercise choices in this book where you don't need to be flat on your back, so why not use them instead?

3. Avoid doing crunches or planks, or being on all fours and other front-loaded positions. There are more details on this in chapter 3, but for now take into consideration that when you turn yourself onto all fours you will have the pull of gravity working against a stretched and compromised core. Crunches put pressure on your compromised

core and create downward pressure on the pelvic floor—not what a pregnant mama needs! Please don't freak out if you are on all fours for a few brief moments, as some of us mamas need to crawl around after our other little kids occasionally. It is repeated and lengthy strains we should protect ourselves against.

4. Listen to your body. If you haven't before, now is the time to really check in with yourself during your workouts. If your body tells you to slow down or stop, don't ignore it. During my two pregnancies I had several workouts where my body told me "This isn't feeling right." So I immediately stopped and either rested or pulled the plug on the workout for that day.

How to Review Your Plan with Your Doctor

Based on the four steps in this framework, make a preliminary plan and then review it with your doctor. If you generally ask, "What should I do about exercise?" then don't be surprised if she provides a very general answer and you're left hanging on the specifics. By showing her what you plan to do and explaining why you are thinking of doing it

that way, you'll have a good dialogue about one of the most powerful preventive measures you can take in your health and your baby's health. You'll also have confidence that you are undertaking something that is safe (and awesome!) for you and baby. Your conversation may look something like this:

"I'm know I am a beginner when it comes to exercise, as I have at most exercised a couple times a week recently (step 1). But I want to be healthy for baby and myself, so I plan to walk or use the elliptical machine for twenty minutes a day to help train my heart and my baby's heart (steps 2 and 3). I won't get too intense, as I will only go at a level where I can carry on a conversation during the workout. I've read that it's important for me to strengthen my core, pelvic floor, glutes, low back, and hips during pregnancy, so I have a few specific exercises for these parts that prenatal experts developed. I'd like to show them to you for your okay. I plan to do these middle part exercises most days (steps 2 and 4). I may even try and to incorporate a couple days of strength training in each trimester with exercises from this book that are designed for each trimester, but I know that because I'm a beginner I will do the beginner option, which is light weights or no weights. I'll be including some prenatal yoga moves from this book (step 4). Let's go over these so we can make sure they are okay for me."

or

"I am really into exercising and consider myself an advanced exerciser; as you know I always get a few workouts in every week (step 1). I will be doing a moderate cardio activity for heart health, like going on the elliptical or walking briskly, nothing high impact so that my pelvic floor is protected. I'll probably do this for thirty minutes every day and I'll ensure that I can carry on a conversation during my workout to keep my intensity in check (steps 2 and 3). Maybe I'll go for a jog once a week because I love running—any objections to that? I have three specific pelvic floor and core exercises that I'll be doing every night before bed; can you take a look at these and give your okay? I'm also game to do some strength training three to five times a week using exercises from this book (steps 2 and 4). I've lifted weights regularly and understand good form. Let's go over these so we can make sure they are okay for me."

As you can see, a fit pregnancy is not done just one way. But being too general leaves us mamas scratching our heads on what can even be done or where our focus should be. This framework can be scaled down or up based on your personal medical situation, but the point is that it gives you something concrete to put into a preliminary plan that you can review with your doctor.

Don't be shy about this. Would you hesitate asking about your precautionary screenings if your doctor didn't bring it up? This is no different. Exercise is an incredibly powerful precaution against many pregnancy-related risks for you and baby, but it needs to be done right for you and your situation. Take control today!

Your Fit First Trimester Nutrition

With a lot of baby-building work to do inside, now is the best time to gain some basic nutrition knowledge. You'll start to look at your food choices a bit differently and see the food's power and purpose in fueling the important work your body is performing over the next nine months. I also want you to be able to avoid the most common traps women fall into when attempting to improve their nutrition. It's frustrating to see women try to "eat better" but instead be tripped up by a few common myths about "healthy foods."

Macronutrients:
The Building Blocks

The concept of *macronutrients* or "macros" is gaining in popularity as a term in dieting and perhaps you've even heard the term; however, when I ask my clients if they know what macros means, 90 percent respond "No" or "Not really." Why would a pregnant woman care about macros? Macronutrients are the first set of building blocks when it comes to nutrition—building blocks for you and building blocks for baby.

Let's start by breaking down the term macronutrients. *Macro* means "large" and *nutrient* means "a substance that provides nourishment essential for growth and maintenance of life." Put those together and *macronutrients* means what you need in large quantities to nourish and grow life. Sounds pretty important! So what specifically are macronutrients? There are three kinds of macros: carbohydrates, proteins, and fats. Yup, you need all three in large quantities to nourish and grow both you and baby.

The dieting industry has messed around with our perception of at least two of the three macronutrients as "low fat" and "low carb" have been woven into dieting protocols over the past few decades. Let's take a close look at each macronutrient so you can see how awesome all three macronutrients are for you and baby.

PROTEIN

This macronutrient is a key source of the amino acids that build your baby's precious toes, button nose, and every cell in between. I put this macronutrient first as my clients too often mistake certain foods as "good sources" of protein when they are actually more of a source of fat and/or carbohydrate. Also, many food packages these days say "High in Protein," but those can be misleading, and I want you to get the real scoop.

There are eight amino acids that we must get from protein, and they are so important that they are called essential amino acids. We need all eight of these every single day because they are essential! Unlike fat and carbohydrates, our body cannot store amino acids, so this means we need to be eating good sources of protein throughout the day, every day.

How much protein a day do you need? It depends on your weight and activity level, but it is well accepted that pregnant women need more protein because it supports growth and development. Most guidelines indicate a pregnant woman should have 70 grams of protein a day, compared to 45 grams for the average woman. However, these guidelines are too general, as they don't take into account your body weight or activity level. Besides, during your pregnancy I would not coach you to weigh and measure your food, so having a hard and fast number is unimportant. A more practical approach, and one I followed in my pregnancy, is to:

1. Be able to identify food sources that are good protein sources.

2. Be able to easily serve yourself an appropriate portion size of that protein source (see Handy Portion Size guidance).

3. Eat a good source of protein in the appropriate portion size at every meal and most snacks (1-2 snacks a day) and you'll be getting enough quality protein to build baby.

How do you know if a food is a good source of protein? If it comes in a container or package, spin it around and see how many grams are listed per serving. If it has 10 grams or more of protein, then it has a decent amount of protein. I've listed some of my top choices of protein below. However, the quality and source of protein matter so I've also described the top three protein traps that women fall into; I want you to avoid these not just in your pregnancy but as part of your approach to healthy and balanced eating.

CARBOHYDRATES

Carbohydrates (aka "carbs") are our energy source, and if there is anything you're probably feeling now, it's a lack of energy. Carbs are broken down to glucose in our bodies and passed along to our baby through the placenta as our shared major fuel source. Yet it's worth noting that overeating carbohydrates, particularly refined and processed carbohydrates, can spike your (and therefore baby's) insulin levels. Just think about a time when you ate a really large, highly refined carbohydrate meal such as Thanksgiving dinner. Remember the energy crash that happened afterward? That was your body spiking glucose and crashing afterward. Repeat this cycle often enough and you raise the risk of many health-related issues for both you and baby, like gestational diabetes.

So how do you balance the energy equation? I love practical approaches to everything nutrition and exercise related—it's the only way we busy gals can make it work! So for this macronutrient I include the same three steps as with protein; however, the main difference is that you should be including a quality carb choice at every snack and meal.

FOOD	SERVING SIZE Refer to Handy Portion photos to easily serve yourself!	PROTEIN
Turkey breast (or extra lean ground turkey)	3.5 ounces	30 g
Salmon	3.5 ounces	26 g
Chicken (no skin)	3.5 ounces	25 g
Lean ground beef	3.5 ounces	25 g
Tuna (water packed)	1/2 can	21 g
Cottage cheese, low fat	1/2 cup	20 g
Greek yogurt, plain low fat	3/4 cup	18 g
Grass-fed New Zealand whey protein (no additives, whey concentrate)	1 scoop	18 g

1. Be able to identify food sources that are good carbohydrate sources. **This means choosing complex carbohydrates as often as you can as your source of carbohydrates. These include whole grains, vegetables, fruits, and legumes. Limit refined carbohydrates like refined flours and sugary junk food.**

2. Be able to easily serve yourself an appropriate portion size **of that carbohydrate source (see Handy Portion Size guidance on page 35).**

3. Eat a good source of carbohydrate in the appropriate portion size at every meal and every snack **(2–3 snacks/day).**

Top 3 Protein Traps

TRAP 1: Greek Yogurt Yumminess: There are a million kinds of Greek yogurt, but too few are "good" choices. This creamy yogurt has soared in popularity in recent years and provides probiotics by the spoonful that help with the many digestive issues we pregnant women experience, like constipation, gas, and bloating. It also is much higher in protein than regular yogurt, as Greek yogurt typically provides 12–18 grams of protein per serving compared to the 4–6 grams in traditional yogurt. This makes Greek yogurt a protein-packed snack, breakfast, or dessert choice. However, along with consumer popularity came dozens of yummy flavors and brands to choose from, and unfortunately few are good choices for baby and mom-to-be. Here's what to watch out for in choosing your Greek yogurt.

SUGAR CRAZE Leave it to food marketers to take a good food source, load it up with sugar, and still package it as "healthy." All of the different flavors of Greek yogurt you see, while sounding (and tasting) delish, often have more sugar in them than a chocolate bar. Read the label and scan the nutritional stats. About 4–6 grams of sugar is naturally occurring in this dairy product; however, most flavored Greek yogurts will pack almost 20 grams of sugar from the flavor added! Instead, choose plain low-fat Greek yogurt and add your own fruit to get that sweet taste and provide baby the nutritional benefits of fruit. I've included several ways to make Greek yogurt yummy and still healthy in the Preggo Power recipes in chapter 7.

ARTIFICIALLY LOADED Does the Greek yogurt you're looking at seem like a good choice because it's low in sugar when you look at the nutrition stats? Check the ingredient listing for artificial sweeteners such as sucralose or acesulfame potassium. Avoid artificial sweeteners, as the impact of these on your baby is not well known.

TRAP 2: Nuts about Nuts and More Peanut Butter Please! Nuts and nut butters are more of a fat than a protein. Most women think they are getting a good dose of protein when they eat almonds or smear on peanut butter (okay, or maybe when they eat peanut butter off the spoon!). While there is some protein in nuts and nut butters, these are more of a fat source than protein source. A small handful of almonds has 15 grams of fat compared to 7 grams of protein, and 1 tablespoon of peanut butter has 8 grams of fat compared to 3 grams of protein. Fat is typically two to three times the protein quantity in nuts and nut butters, so it makes more sense to look at nuts as a healthy fat macronutrient instead of protein. There are many better sources of protein; just check out the list above. A piece of chicken at 25 grams of protein a serving doesn't even compare to that spoonful of peanut butter at 3 grams.

TRAP 3: Packaged Protein Products: When I first because familiar with macronutrients I was drawn to products that said right on the package, "Good Source of Protein!" Cereals, breads, bars, and drinks. I thought, *Cool! An easy way to get in some more protein*. As I became more educated about the sources of protein, I was shocked to find out that almost every packaged protein product in my grocery store used soy as the protein source. So what? Soy is a controversial topic. On one hand, you have people listing the health benefits—it's low in calories and a complete source of protein (maybe), and it can help reduce cholesterol and heart disease. On the other hand, there are too many studies to ignore that soy can be quite detrimental to your health. In particular, soy can interfere with your hormone balance and contribute to premature puberty, and it has been linked to certain types of cancer. Messing with hormones in a pregnant woman (or any woman) raises a red flag for me—and so I recommend that all my clients avoid all soy-based products, especially the processed soy found in packaged cereals, breads, bars, and drinks.

To add some context to the prevalent use of soy in packaged foods, soy is a cheap source of protein, so it's not a surprise that soy is the choice of protein for food corporations so they can slap on a "High Protein" label and capture more sales from unaware consumers. That may sound cynical, but profit-driven companies have bottom lines to manage and don't always have your health on the top of their priority list.

Below are a few of my favorite carb sources during pregnancy that also include lots of vitamins and mineral benefits for baby and are also good sources of fiber. I grouped them into categories to help you become familiar with the appropriate portion sizes. In particular, notice how a portion of fruit is less than a portion vegetables? Fruits are more carbohydrate dense as well as high in natural sugars. Fruits are good for you, but you don't need as large of a portion to get the carbs you need to fuel you and baby.

One thing that may surprise you is finding low-fat dairy under carbs. Few people think of dairy products as a source of carbohydrates; however, due to the naturally occurring lactose sugar in milk, dairy products are often as much if not more of a source of carbohydrates than protein. A glass of skim milk has 12 grams of carbs and 8 grams of protein—that's 1.5 times as many carbs as protein! Low-fat plain Greek yogurt has 12 grams of carbs and 18 grams of protein, so while Greek yogurt is an awesome source of protein, you are also getting quality carbs with that snack.

FATS

We've become comfortable with the benefits of including healthy fats in our diets. Most of us can easily identify good fats like raw nuts,

HAVE YOUR FILL CARBS	BE MINDFUL CARBS	KEEP IT IN CHECK CARBS
Veggies (Non-starchy) Examples: kale, broccoli, spinach, cucumber, asparagus, peppers	**Fruit** Examples: small apple, small pear, 1 cup berries, 1 cup grapes, banana	**Grains & Starchy Veggies** Examples: 1/2 cup cooked brown rice, 1/2 cup sweet potatoes, 1/2 cup uncooked plain oatmeal, 1 cup carrots, 1 slice whole wheat bread, 1 small wrap
	Low-fat Dairy Examples: 8 ounces skim milk, 3/4 cup Greek yogurt	

avocado, olive oil, nut butters, and coconut oil. We want to include three to four servings a day of the good fats in our diet during our pregnancy. Omega-3 fatty acids, particularly DHA, are awesome for baby because DHA is needed for proper brain growth and eye development in your baby. Many of the Preggo Power recipes in this book include foods rich in DHA such as salmon, walnuts, chicken, and flaxseed. You may also want to discuss including a DHA supplement with your doctor.

While it's great that so many women are no longer shy about including fats in their diets, I find that most women don't have their portion sizes nailed for this important macronutrient. Many clients are shocked at how easily they go over their daily fat requirement, as the portion sizes they are doling out are too large. Fats are the most energy-dense macronutrient, packing 9 calories per gram of fat compared to 4 calories per gram of carbs and protein. You need less than half a serving of fats to fuel you and baby! Take the time to review the Handy Portion Sizes guide (see page 36) for your favorite fat sources to ensure that fats are fueling, not fattening, you.

Handy Portion Sizes and Calories

During your first trimester, there is no need for your calorie intake to increase unless you are currently underweight. Your doctor will give you guidelines for increasing or decreasing your calories if you need to, so be sure to ask! But for those in a healthy pre-pregnancy weight range, the first trimester is best used as an opportunity to remind us of our portion sizes to keep our pregnancy weight gain within the healthy range of 25–35 pounds.

The following Handy Portion Sizes guide shows you what a sensible portion size for each macronutrient looks like using your hands. The cool thing about your hands is that you take them everywhere! You have the portion-control tool you need everywhere you go, including restaurants, your in-laws' house, and your own kitchen.

Food Aversions and Nausea

If you're feeling queasy just looking at some of the food portion photos, then I feel for you. I spent the better part of three months during my first trimester feeling like I was hungover. I held my breath when I opened the fridge door to avoid smelling the food, and after one morning's puking episode I checked into the hospital

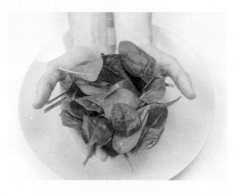

TWO LARGE HANDFULS

Fill up your plate with any non-starchy vegetable, like salad, green beans, or cucumbers. Starchy vegetables like carrots, potatoes, and sweet potatoes should have a smaller portion, as shown below. Remember these are plain veggies, so if you add any sauces or oils, they follow their own portion-control guidelines.

ONE LARGE HANDFUL

Starchy vegetables, like carrots and sweet potatoes, are good for you, but should be enjoyed in a smaller portion than non-starchy vegtables. Why? These guys have a much higher carbohydrate content than those leafy greens. For example, one handful of sweet potatoes has 20 grams of carbs compared to less than 2 grams of carbs in two handfuls of spinach.

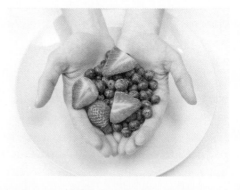

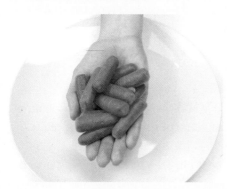

Fruit is also great for you, as it's a delicious way to get you and baby the nutrients you both need to thrive. However, the sugar and carbohydrate content is much higher in fruit than in vegetables, so enjoy these with portion parameters in mind. I too often see my coworkers scarfing massive bowls of fruit salad (like massive!) at their desk in an attempt to eat healthier. However, the sugar and carbs in the too-big portion sends their energy crashing soon after. One handful of fruit typically has 15–20 grams of carbs and usually at least 10 grams of sugar. While the sugar is natural, it is still sugar, so a bit of moderation here is important.

OPEN PALM

Lean, mean protein! For women I often find that the portions chosen of this macronutrient are not enough. Your protein portions from lean sources like chicken, lean ground turkey, and fish should cover the entire palm of your hand. Even enjoying lean ground beef, bison, and fatty fish once a week in this portion is great for you and baby.

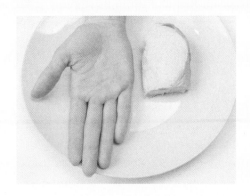

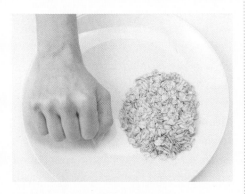

ONE FIST/KEPT IN CHECK

Grains are great for you and your baby! In particular, whole grains like oatmeal and whole wheat bread are an important source of many nutrients, including fiber, B vitamins, folate, and minerals. However, these can quickly get out of control as plates are loaded with pasta and rice, and bread comes by the basket! One fist or one small slice is a sensible serving of 20–25 grams of carbohydrates.

GOOD IN SMALL DOSES

Healthy fats have become well accepted because they have amazing nutrition benefits, like better brain function and improved skin and eye health. However, the portion size of one serving of these healthy fats often shocks my clients. Just 12–16 almonds is a serving. Next time, count out those nuts, then look at the scant handful in your palm. Yup, that's it. Most people are eating nuts by the large mittful (after mittful)! Nut butters and healthy oils like olive oil are similar—a spoonful is all you need.

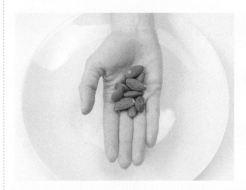

with dehydration. The only foods that I could stomach were plain crackers, soup, and bagels for most of my first trimester. Trying to eat specific foods because they are good for you and baby is a ridiculous piece of advice when you're feeling this way, so I chose low-sodium soups and crackers and whole wheat bagels with low-fat cream cheese. Honestly, if someone held up a piece of chicken and veggies at me, I may have thrown it back at them! Fortunately, that nausea passed and I made good nutrition choices, more often than not, in my second and third trimesters. That's two out of three trimesters, and I did the best I could during the nausea and food aversions—I call that a win!

Notice how I didn't have an all-or-nothing mentality? I didn't say to myself, *Oh well, since I can't eat Preggo Power foods, I'll just eat as much junk as I want,* or *Why bother starting now?* when I started to feel better. It's never too late to turn it around, as your baby is developing not just in one day but over all three trimesters! Start today with just a few better choices and aim to consistently choose better most of the time instead of being unrealistic and aiming for perfection.

Preggo Power Vitamins and Minerals

We know our food choices aren't perfect, and even if we're nailing our nutrition, our food sources can lack the vitamins and minerals we need to support healthy development for baby. This section shines the spotlight on the key ones. However, excessive amounts of certain nutrients can also be hazardous, so don't pop pills, thinking that more is better. Plan your vitamins and review the plan with your doctor like you would any medication. It would be difficult to overdose on the vitamins and minerals through the foods you are eating, but it's the extra supplements or vitamin-fortified packaged foods and drinks that can pose a risk if not reviewed.

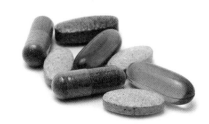

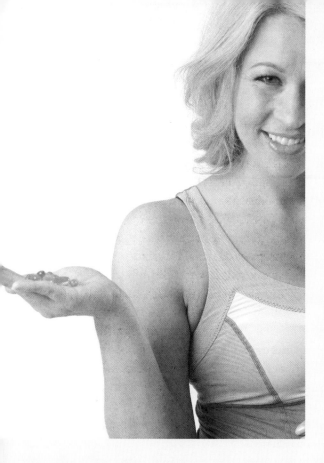

risk of neural tube defects like spina bifida in your baby. Therefore this is one vitamin you'll want to specifically ensure you are getting enough of daily (400–600 micrograms).

IRON

During pregnancy, your iron requirements increase to support the development of your baby's blood cells. An iron supplement is commonly needed in addition to a prenatal vitamin; however, many stores keep iron behind the pharmacy counter to ensure that the customer knows the correct dosage, as too much iron can harm baby. Be sure to talk to your doctor about recommended dosage.

Timing of this mineral can be one of the trickiest, as it's most effective when paired with vitamin C for best absorption, yet iron should be avoided with calcium-rich foods or if your prenatal vitamin has calcium in it, because calcium interferes with iron absorption.

DHA

An essential fat found primarily in fish, this specific fat gets the spotlight because of its ability to improve brain health for baby. If fish isn't your favorite, then review taking a DHA supplement with your doctor.

PRENATAL VITAMINS

While it's standard practice to take a prenatal vitamin, there unfortunately are no standards for prenatal vitamins. Some prenatal vitamins include DHA, while others do not. The amount of folic acid varies widely between brands. Some prenatal vitamins can even include herbs you may want to avoid. So be sure to check with your doctor before selecting your prenatal vitamin.

FOLIC ACID

Studies show that taking a vitamin containing folic acid before pregnancy as well as in the first few months of pregnancy significantly reduces the

Can I Take Protein Powder?

We are wary of taking some mystery powder stuff. Is protein powder safe for baby? This again is an "it depends" answer, and if at the end of this section and after chatting with your doctor you're still uncertain, then be cautious and avoid using anything you are unsure of during pregnancy.

The main points to consider in deciding if you want to take a protein powder while pregnant:

1. Supplements, including protein powders, are not required to get US Food and Drug Administration (FDA) approval. This means that many protein powders have never been reviewed for their ingredients before they go to market. Unlike drug products, which must be proven safe and effective for their intended use before marketing, there are no provisions in the law for FDA to approve dietary supplements for safety or effectiveness before they reach the consumer.

   The FDA will take action if complaints are brought to its attention; however, you want to protect baby before the FDA gets involved. Your confidence in the manufacturer's quality-control and ingredient list must be rock solid. At a minimum, go to the company's website and see if they talk about their quality-control processes—you'll find that few do, which is telling of the quality of most supplements in the market.

2. Read the label carefully and avoid protein powders with artificial sweeteners and other mystery ingredients. Protein powders that are marketed to athletes and bodybuilders might contain ingredients that are not safe for you and baby. Avoiding artificial sweeteners, such as saccharin, aspartame, and sucralose, is a good idea at any time, but especially during pregnancy. The safest approach is to take a protein that is naturally flavored, which means it is labeled as being sweetened with fructose (fruit sugar) or stevia.

3. Just protein? Most protein powders are high in protein but low in carbohydrates and fats. To make it a complete meal, you would need to eat more food with it or add ingredients into the blender such as fruit (carbs), almond butter (fat), spinach, and so on. Some protein powders have a balance of protein, carbs, and fats as well as fiber to replicate a meal. You'll need to read the nutritional statistics on the label to see if the protein powder you're looking at is just protein or more of a meal replacement. A meal replacement protein powder would have approximately 26–36 grams of protein, 20–30 grams of carbs, 6–10 grams of fat, and a healthy dose of fiber (anything over 3 grams of fiber is good). Compare that to a simple protein powder, which typically has 26–36 grams of protein but less than 2 grams of carbs or fats.

I did take a high-quality meal replacement type of protein powder during my pregnancy, as I found it an easy and convenient way to get in the important balance of macronutrients we mommies-to-be need. I'd sip a berry meal replacement shake in the morning while getting myself and my family out the door before work. In the afternoon I'd shake up a chocolate meal-type of shake while also noshing on some cut veggies. I'd still eat two additional meals plus snacks each day, but with the food aversions I experienced in the first trimester, it was a good solution for me to have a better balance of quality macronutrients. For the supplement brand that I felt comfortable using during my pregnancy, you can visit my website at www.sisinshape.com and click on Shop.

Preggo Power Foods Meal Planner and Sample Menu: First Trimester

Even if you're feeling as if there is no way you could stomach anything beyond a box of crackers, take a peek at this first trimester menu and you might be surprised how good nutrition can also be tummy-friendly. Choosing just a few more nutrient-dense options is a great start to fueling your baby's growth and development.

Feeling tired? Getting up for work

Breakfast:

CHOOSE ONE OF:

- Fruit-Filled Overnight Quinoa & Oats
- Carrot Cake Overnight Oats
- Breakfast Muesli Bowl
- Protein smoothie that has all macro-nutrients (look for high-quality meal replacement type or add in fats and carbohydrates such as almond butter, banana, and a handful of spinach).

Snack Mid-Morning and Late Afternoon:

CHOOSE ONE FOR EACH MID-MORNING AND LATE AFTERNOON SNACK:

- Blackberry Maple Almond Butter Greek Yogurt
- PBJ Protein Bars
- Hardboiled egg and an apple
- 16–24 almonds (1–1.5 servings of nuts) and a serving of fruit

Lunch & Dinner:

ANY OF THE POWER PREGGO LUNCH/DINNER RECIPES (SEE PAGE 164) *PLUS* 1 SERVING OF COMPLEX CARBOHYDRATES (WHOLE WHEAT BREAD, BROWN RICE, ETC.). EACH RECIPE IS PACKED WITH BABY-BUILDING NUTRIENTS.

- Build a meal that is well balanced with sources of protein, carbohydrates, and fat. Load up on veggies for an extra power boost.

- The Handy Portion Size guide helps you choose an infinite number of food options yet keeps those portions in check in a simple way.

in the morning was a big struggle for me in the first trimester, so I found simple yet healthy breakfast solutions. Have you ever tried overnight oats? This is a breakfast you can easily make the night before and just heat up in the morning. If you can't eat first thing in the morning due to nausea, these easy breakfast options also travel well. Take breakfast with you in a container to nosh on when your stomach is feeling ready.

You'll notice the rest of the snacks and meals are well balanced with all three macronutrients and were also selected because they are packed with baby-building nutrients!

Your Fit First Trimester Workouts

This first trimester workout program is designed to create the foundation of a strong body from head to toe. Therefore the focus of this program is on maintaining and even increasing your strength and flexibility. Each workout will take you approximately 30 minutes to complete. There are no high-impact moves, as relaxin levels are at their highest during the first trimester.

In your first trimester:

Incorporate at least three Core Confidence moves at least five times a week (refer to chapter 3).

Go for an additional 20–30 minute walk or choose a low-impact cardio activity if your schedule permits.

YOUR FIT FIRST TRIMESTER						
Day 1	Day 2	Day 3	Day 4	Day 5	Day 6	Day 7
Strength Train: Legs	Cardio Activity	Strength Train: Shoulders Focus	Strength Train: Chest + Back	Yoga / Stretch	Strength Train: Arms Focus	Cardio Activity
Include at least three Core Confidence moves five times a week (chapter 3).						
If your schedule permits, add an additional 20–30 minutes of walking or low-impact cardio activity.						

STRENGTH TRAINING

The Basics

For each exercise, choose a weight that ensures you are not straining or compromising your form at any point during the exercise.

Keep progressing in your first trimester! If you could easily perform five more repetitions, then consider increasing the weight for the next set. However, never strain yourself to complete a repetition.

Rest between sets. Take adequate rest in between each set to ensure that you could easily carry on a normal conversation while exercising. This may be as little as 30 seconds or up to a couple minutes of rest.

This program's exercises are to be completed superset style, which means you complete exercise 1 for the prescribed number of reps then immediately perform exercise 2 before taking a rest. You then repeat exercise A1+A2 (or B1+B2, etc.) for the prescribed number of sets.

Stop exercising if you feel you are pushing it. Some days are like that—always listen to your body.

BEGINNER: Complete 1–2 sets of each exercise for 12–15 repetitions. Choose a light weight or use your own body weight. For exercises that indicate the use of a barbell, substitute a resistance band with handles to perform the movement.

Finish your workout with a 15-minute walk or elliptical session.

INTERMEDIATE: Complete 2–3 sets of each exercise for 12–15 repetitions.

If performing 2 sets, then finish your workout with a 15-minute walk or elliptical session.

ADVANCED: Complete 3–4 sets of each exercise for 10–12 repetitions. The repetitions are fewer than for the intermediate as it is assumed that you are choosing a heavier weight yet still executing the moves with excellent form.

DAY 1—STRENGTH TRAIN: LEGS

A1	A2	B1	B2	C1	C2
Leg extension (toes straight)	Step-ups on bench	**BEGINNER:** Squat (body weight only)	Calf raises (toes straight)	**BEGINNER:** Cable pull-through*	Calf raises (toes out)
		INT/ADV: Squat*		**INT/ADV:** Deadlift*	

*Only if you have excellent form. Keep weight light to avoid straining or pushing through pelvic area.

DAY 3—STRENGTH TRAIN: SHOULDERS FOCUS

A1	A2	B1	B2	C1	C2
Arnold press	Cable woodchop	Plate landmine	Seated shoulder press	BOSU preggo "burpee"	Leaning side lateral raise

DAY 4—STRENGTH TRAIN: CHEST + BACK

A1	A2	B1	B2	C1	C2
Parallel-grip lat pull-down	Incline chest press	Single-arm row on bench	Incline chest flye	Reverse-grip lat pull-down	Hands-out push-up

DAY 6—STRENGTH TRAIN: ARMS FOCUS

A1	A2	B1	B2	C1	C2
Hammer curl	Tricep dip on bench	Side plank	Tricep rope extension	21s	Bird dog

CARDIO

The Basics:

Choose a low-impact activity that raises your heart rate slightly for 20–30 minutes while ensuring that you can easily carry on a normal conversation while exercising.

The activity does not need to be performed for a continuous 30 minutes. Two 15-minute sessions are equally as effective.

Remember that you are getting in cardiovascular benefits for you and baby during your strength training sessions, too!

Activity options for Days 2 and 7:

- Walking
- Elliptical machine
- Stepper machine
- Swimming
- Stationary bike

YOGA

This yoga-based sequence of five prenatal stretches and restorative poses takes you from standing to sitting to lying down.

Hold or gently move through each pose for 2–3 minutes, focusing on your breath.

Breathe slowly in and out through your nose.

Gently move your body through the full range of motion, never straining during a pose.

Repeat the sequence for a total of two sequences.

DAY 5—YOGA / STRETCH				
1	2	3	4	5
L-standing supported by wall	Cat/cow	Spinal balance pose	Seated straddle twist	Child pose

PREGGO PAL PROFILE Katy Livingstone

"Being a Different Kind of Fit"

THIS IS MY SECOND BABY (both boys), and nothing about my two pregnancies has been similar. I had no morning sickness, barely any pains and strains, and was very active with baby number 1, who was delivered naturally. This time around, I've had morning sickness, headaches, pubic symphysis dysfunction, and placenta previa, meaning I will be delivering via C-section. My activity level went from swinging kettlebells and running 10K races during my first pregnancy to barely being able to walk the second time around!

I can't say it hasn't been frustrating. I am a high school physical educator, and it has been really hard to slow down. I really want to be an example to the teenage girls I teach, letting them know it's not only okay but advisable to be active. I have been forced to slow down and focus on being fit from a recovery standpoint. Daily activities such as walking and stair climbing—though painful—fill my fitness quota, and pelvic floor exercises are my new staple. This will hopefully make my recovery faster and enable me to rekindle my love of fitness when my body heals. I just don't know when that will be.

I have all these ideas in my head of what I would like to do—complete another duathlon, run a 5K with my baby—will that be attainable? I'm not sure. Add it to the list of pregnant woman worries!

> You can connect with Katy on all things fitness and fashion on her public social media profiles: Facebook "Fit in Heels" and Twitter/Instagram @ fit_in_heels.

MY FIT BUMP

FIRST TRIMESTER (4 WEEKS)

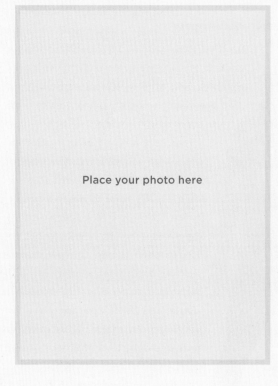

Place your photo here

MY FIT BUMP

FIRST TRIMESTER (8 WEEKS)

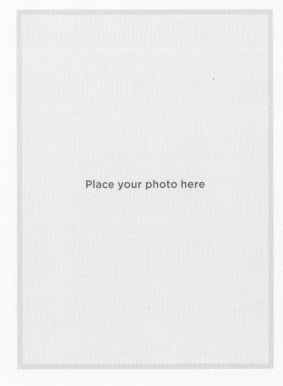

Place your photo here

MY FIT BUMP

FIRST TRIMESTER (12 WEEKS)

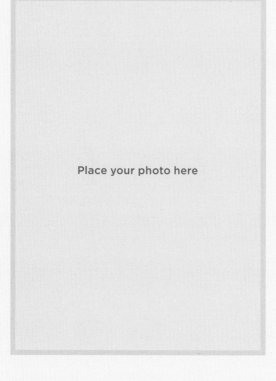

Place your photo here

I AM A "BODYBUILDER"

Right now, I am the world's most natural bodybuilder. I am literally building a body inside of me!

I AM STRENGTHING...

My arms, so I can _____ with you.

My heart, so I can _____ with you.

My legs, so I can _____ with you.

My mind, so I can _____ with you.

> "My body is full of life.
> My body is powerful.
> My body made me a mother."
>
> —UNKNOWN

MY FIT FIRST TRIMESTER | NUTRITION

MY TYPICAL DAILY MENU

Breakfast _____
_____

❑ Water

Mid-morning _____
_____

❑ Water

Lunch _____
_____

❑ Water

Mid-afternoon _____
_____

❑ Water

Dinner _____
_____

❑ Water

Evening (optional) _____
_____

❑ Water

MY FIT FIRST TRIMESTER | NUTRITION
SHOPPING LIST

Lean Proteins
- ❑ _____
- ❑ _____
- ❑ _____
- ❑ _____

Complex Carbs
- ❑ _____
- ❑ _____
- ❑ _____
- ❑ _____

Fruits & Veggies
- ❑ _____
- ❑ _____
- ❑ _____
- ❑ _____

Healthy Fats
- ❑ _____
- ❑ _____
- ❑ _____
- ❑ _____

MY FIT FIRST TRIMESTER

EXERCISE & TRACKING SHEET

EXERCISE NAME	MONTH 1 (REPS & LBS)	MONTH 2 (REPS & LBS)	MONTH 3 (REPS & LBS)

CORE CONFIDENCE TRACKER:

Put a checkmark below each time you strengthen your core & pelvic floor.

❏ ❏ ❏ ❏ ❏ ❏ ❏ ❏ ❏ ❏ ❏ ❏

CARDIO

Note your cardio activity this trimester:

_____

_____

MY FIT FIRST TRIMESTER

EXERCISE & TRACKING SHEET

EXERCISE NAME	MONTH 1 (REPS & LBS)	MONTH 2 (REPS & LBS)	MONTH 3 (REPS & LBS)

CORE CONFIDENCE TRACKER:

Put a checkmark below each time you strengthen your core & pelvic floor.

❑ ❑ ❑ ❑ ❑ ❑ ❑ ❑ ❑ ❑ ❑ ❑

CARDIO

Note your cardio activity this trimester:

_____

_____

_____

MY FIT FIRST TRIMESTER

EXERCISE & TRACKING SHEET

EXERCISE NAME	MONTH 1 (REPS & LBS)	MONTH 2 (REPS & LBS)	MONTH 3 (REPS & LBS)

CORE CONFIDENCE TRACKER:

Put a checkmark below each time you strengthen your core & pelvic floor.

☐ ☐ ☐ ☐ ☐ ☐ ☐ ☐ ☐ ☐ ☐ ☐

CARDIO

Note your cardio activity this trimester:

_____

_____

_____

Notes: _____
_____
_____
_____
_____
_____
_____
_____
_____
_____
_____
_____
_____
_____
_____
_____
_____
_____
_____
_____
_____
_____
_____
_____
_____
_____
_____
_____
_____

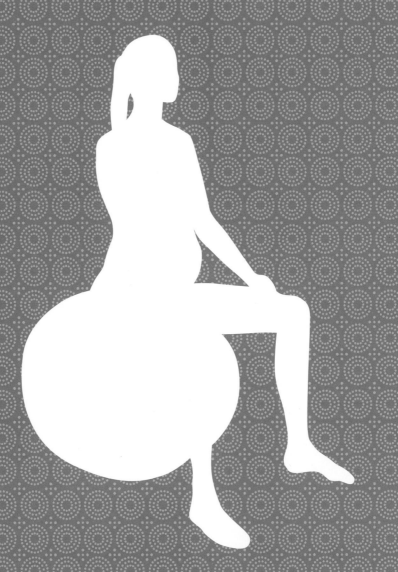

CORE CONFIDENCE AND PELVIC FLOOR POWER

→ The first cradle baby has is your core. Let's create a healthy place for her while she's there and a functional one for you after!

Sister to sister, this part needs full honesty. Your middle parts are going to go through hell over the next nine months. They will be stretched and strained, and may even tear. Your abs, pelvic floor, glutes, hips, and low back surround, cradle, and support that adorable little baby bump. They are also critical in your ability to move, lift, dance, make love, pick up baby for a cuddle, as well as haul around the massive amounts of laundry guaranteed to be in your future. Your middle parts also ensure that you pee when you should and not when you shouldn't. Talk about important! Yet, the number one fitness question I get from pregnant women is "Can I do abs?" They fear harming baby, as the only ab exercise they can think of is a crunch, and who wants to crunch their baby? Some also think that since they are guaranteed to *not* get a six-pack over the next nine months, they don't see the point of ab work. Without the right information and at a loss for what actually to do, most women avoid exercising all of their middle parts during the time they need the most attention.

Can I Even Do Abs? *Pre*habilitiation of Your Core

Not many woman know about this area because no one talks to pregnant women about bladder leaks, separated abs (called diastasis recti), and even the possibility that your uterus could slip down into your vaginal canal or even fall out postpartum. (*Excuse me, my uterus can go where?* you ask. It's called prolapse, and more on that in a moment.) While everyone seems willing to give sleeping, feeding, and parenting advice to pregnant moms, why not discuss this?

Unfortunately, not many women, or even health and fitness professionals, for that matter, know the intricacies of the pelvic floor and core to know how to best support it during pregnancy as well as afterward to help avoid the myriad problems that can occur postpartum from the physical stress of childbearing and delivery.

Also our popular approaches to six-pack abs (crunch, sit-up, repeat) actually contribute to making our poor stretched-out, even damaged, tummies worse. Well, yay you! Because you're preggo you're actually in the best place possible right now to do the right exercises to prevent pelvic floor problems and core crises postpartum. As the ladies say at Bellies Inc., "It is much easier to prepare than repair."

Bellies Inc. on a Mission to Eliminate "Mummy Tummy"

Bellies Inc. was founded by three experts in the area of pre- and postnatal fitness and physiotherapy in 2010. These three women came together with the vision of more effective and innovative strategies for core health during pregnancy, as well as for new moms. The founders heard too many of their clients and patients say, "Why did no one tell me this before?" when they explained that the postpartum complications they now faced—like prolapse, incontinence, back pain, and more— could have been prevented with the right pre- and postnatal exercises and systems. Bellies Inc. founders Kim Vopni, Julia Di Paolo, and Samantha Montpetit-Huynh each brought her professional experience and coupled it with the most current scientific research on core health to create an innovative core program and system to help pregnant women prepare their middle for birth and teach them how to optimize their postpartum healing. A surprising spin-off of their work is that they are providing education for fitness professionals and physiotherapists through their certification programs, as too few are in the know when it comes to pelvic floor dysfunction, diastasis (remember, separate abs?), and core *pre*hab and rehab.

The Power of Your Pelvic Floor

Kim and Julia explained to me: "The pelvic floor is part of the core—*it is the foundation*—and it plays a vital role in our everyday movement, yet it doesn't receive a lot of attention, mainly because we can't see it and also because it is a 'taboo' area of the body for many. The pelvic floor is a network of muscles, ligaments, and connective tissue that supports the spine and pelvis and helps keep our internal organs in place."

Picture your growing uterus and the load it is putting on your pelvic floor, the foundation of your core. Add in posture changes (you know you don't stand the same!) and hormonal changes that loosen your ligaments, and your pelvic floor is in need of some serious TLC! Julia adds, "During a vaginal birth, the muscles and nerves of the pelvic floor will be stretched, feel intense pressure, and may become injured. During a C-section birth, the connective tissue involved in the network of the pelvic floor will be cut and surgically repaired, leaving scar tissue. Any of these issues can impact the function of the pelvic floor after baby is born, and the mom may then face an uphill battle as she tries to restore and rebuild her core."

The result of this weakened or damaged pelvic floor could be pelvic floor dysfunction, in which the new mommy experiences incontinence (peeing when you shouldn't), pelvic pain, and prolapse (progressive descent of the internal organs like the bladder, the rectum, and the uterus). So let's get that pelvic floor strong *now* while you're still pregnant and *pre*habilitate this powerful part of your core. How? I'm going to take you beyond Kegels to do this thanks to the ladies at Bellies Inc.

Mummy Tummy

Mummy tummy is the term the Bellies Inc. team applies to a condition called diastasis recti, which is a separation of the rectus abdominis muscles. *Diastasis* means "separation" in Latin. Mummy tummy is characterized by that poochy tummy that too many of us moms try to correct post-baby with endless sit-ups and boot camps. However, mummy tummy cannot be improved with crunches or boot camps—unfortunately, these can actually make the diastasis worse! Even world-class athletes

and avid fitness fanatics who do the wrong type of ab exercises (and never even had babies) can develop diastasis over time.

Julia explains that it's not the "ab gap" that is actually the problem for mummy tummy; instead "it is the stretching and weakening of the linea alba—the connective tissue that is designed to hold the two rectus abdominis muscles in place. The stretching and weakening of the linea alba leads to its inability to generate tension down that middle line of your abdomen which holds the two rectus muscles in place."

A little anatomy lesson will help all this make sense as well as drive home why the right pre/post core work is important. Don't worry, I'll keep it simple!

RECTUS ABODMINIS: You have two halves to your rectus abdominis, a left side and a right side. These start way down at your pelvis and run up to just under your breasts.

LINEA ALBA: The two halves of your rectus abdominis are usually an inch apart and are connected by the fibrous linea alba. Posture, forward pressure, and your growing uterus and the hormone relaxin cause the linea alba to relax, which allows the muscles to move aside for

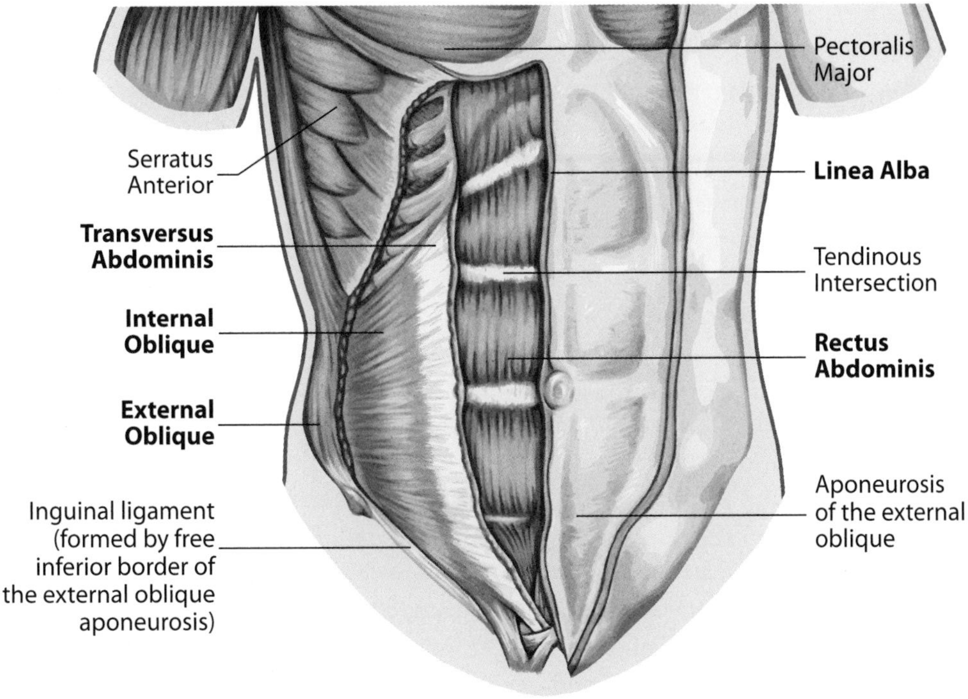
Pectoralis Major
Serratus Anterior
Linea Alba
Transversus Abdominis
Tendinous Intersection
Internal Oblique
Rectus Abdominis
External Oblique
Aponeurosis of the external oblique
Inguinal ligament (formed by free inferior border of the external oblique aponeurosis)

fetal growth, stretch sideways, and become thinner. This is where diastasis occurs.

A cool thing about your linea albea, which in Latin means "white line," is that you can often see it pigmented on your skin during/after pregnancy. It's that dark line running down the middle of your tummy. This pigmented line is called linea nigra ("black line"). Before pregnancy it was likely the same color as your skin; however, because of the increased production of melanin, the linea darkens during pregnancy and usually stays that way for several months following baby's arrival. It's almost as if the body is saying, "Pay attention to me!"

TRANSVERSE ABDOMINIS: Notice in the picture how the transverse abs are the inner layer of the abdominal section? Your transverse abs act as a corset to keep everything tight and support your internal organs. Imagine your transverse abs as a rubber band that's been used (and reused) during pregnancy. After a baby (or two or three) this rubber band gets stretched out, and we're left with a front pooch that sit-ups can't address. Crunches and sit-ups work your rectus abdominals, not your transverse abs—we need to "strengthen from the inside out to abolish mummy tummy!" says Samantha from Bellies Inc.

Strong from the Inside Out

My favorite exercises from Bellies Inc. are described at the end of this chapter and included in this chapter's summary of what to do (or don't) on page 71. You may wonder how some of the exercises flatten your tummy, because they look nothing like the typical core exercises that you have been doing up until now. I come from a fitness background, and I was skeptical if I would find these core exercises challenging enough. Yet as I became more educated about the intricacies of my pregnant core, the Bellies Inc. approach made complete sense! The key to a strong tummy is to work the inner core as a team and encourage the upward motion of the pelvic floor and the inward motion of the transversus abdominus—remember, your innermost abdominal muscle? It is this inward motion of the deep abdominals that helps realign or prevent your abs from separating, and keeps your inner ab band

(tranverse abs) strong and tight! As Kim explains, "The deep abdominals are best activated by first engaging the pelvic floor. You learn how to activate your pelvic floor with your Core Breath, and then you learn how to add it into movement to really get your inner core fired up!"

I put this all to the test, and wow—after the first session did I get a wake-up call! Not only could I tell I was working the right spots, it also showed me how weak this part of my physique was from my first pregnancy. My pelvic floor and abs felt tired and really worked in ways they never had before. I considered myself very fit and was humbled when a restorative breathing technique blasted away my perceived strength in this area.

Upgrade Your Kegel

Let's look at the famous Kegel and talk about why there may be a better way to exercise and strengthen your pelvic floor. This is *Your Fit Pregnancy*, so let's upgrade your pelvic floor fitness! At best, a pregnant woman may know to Kegel to strengthen her pelvic floor, and so she does this at stoplights and grocery store lines. *Squeeeeze your va-jay-jay, hold, release. Squeeeeze, hold, release.* Right? Well, according to the Bellies Inc. team, doing Kegels is not always the best choice. And as a gal who personally Kegeled through her first pregnancy, and then started using the Core Breath technique for baby #2, the ability to actually *feel* the work on my pelvic floor with the Core Breath was awesome.

Remember how your pelvic floor will make sure you don't pee your pants, hold in your internal organs as the foundation of your core, and let you get sexy with your partner (and feel it)? All of these are very important functions for a woman, so let's functionally train our pelvic floor *now* while you're pregnant, when you need it most! And post-baby, you'll be a pro at pelvic floor fitness and will be able to recover faster and stronger with the same exercises.

Julia explains: "Most women often use the wrong muscles in a Kegel. They typically use their glutes and/or their inner thighs. And even if a woman is able to identify the correct muscles, it's not just squeezing that is needed to develop pelvic floor strength. It's squeezing a relaxed and lengthened pelvic floor as well as lifting up your pelvic floor that is needed." It's why most Kegels are ineffective, because the posture of most women sitting at a desk or in a car trying to Kegel is one of a "slouch" or a tucked-in tailbone. All that slouching in our posture shortens our pelvic floor, and if a muscle is already shortened, then contracting a muscle to contract and shorten it more doesn't work! As Julia further explains, "What is needed is a chance to let go and lengthen."

The cool thing about the Core Breath is that you position yourself properly to start and visualize opening your pelvic floor with each breath so the muscle actually has a chance to relax. Julia coaches, "We offer clients some visualization tools to help them find and activate the pelvic floor, cues like: pick up a blueberry with your vagina and your anus as you exhale, and then let the blueberries go as you inhale. Pick up, but don't crush, those blueberries! Or, think about lifting your perineum up to the crown of your head as you exhale and then letting it come back down as you inhale."

Core Confidence Exercises

These are three of my favorite exercises that the gals from Bellies Inc. are letting me share with you! Bellies Inc. developed eight exercises that are great for pre- and postnatal core prehabilitation and rehabilitation.

To get all eight exercises with video demonstrations developed by Bellies Inc., visit my website www.sisinshape.com.

As amazing as these exercises are, one size never fits all. If you have any complications in your pregnancy, the ladies from Bellies Inc., in addition to your doctor, are a great resource for your questions about whether these exercises are right for you. Let them know that you are looking at their Core Breath exercises and that while some of these exercises may be okay, others may not be, so you're looking for their input.

You'll notice I wrote these three exercises into every day of the *Your Fit Pregnancy* program. Yes, I advocate doing all of them every day, or at minimum five times a week. You don't have to do them in the gym or all at once. I put an exercise mat and ball at the foot of my bed as a trigger for me to do my important core work before I got into my comfy bed each night. These exercises are just as important as brushing your teeth, so establish these exercises as a habit by including them into your daily routine. Explain to your partner what you are doing and ask him to support your taking 10 minutes each night to *pre*habilitate your core and pelvic floor. I also found that the Core Breath helped to relax my mind and

prepare me for sleep. If you're doing the breathing correctly, you will find you are somewhat noisy doing these exercises, and thus I felt most comfortable doing these in the privacy of my own home. I also had difficulty focusing properly on these exercises at the gym as the pumping background music and other gym-goers' presence made it challenging for me to close my eyes and visualize picking up berries with my va-jay-jay!

As I mastered the Core Breath, I looked for other opportunities to add this foundational move into my other exercises. It became second nature to fill up my diaphragm and rib cage with air, open and relax my pelvic floor, and then blooooooow out through pursed lips pulling in and up the depths of my core, including my pelvic floor.

Exercise 1: The Core Breath

The Core Breath is both preventive and restorative. What does that mean? During pregnancy the Core Breath will help your core maintain its strength and integrity. Postpartum, it is the first exercise you will do in the early days after your baby's birth to help regenerate tone, strength, and function in your inner core.

A video of the Core Breath is on my YouTube channel under the "Pregnancy Fitness" playlist. The link to my YouTube channel is at www.sisinshape.com.

Here are step-by-step instructions for mastering the Core Breath:

1. Sit on an exercise ball and pull your bum flesh out from under you so you can really feel the sit bones. Your reference points should be your two sit bones and your perineum on the surface of the ball (your "tripod"). Your feet will be flat on the floor and slightly wider than pelvis width apart.

   TIP: Right after having baby, the thought of sitting on a ball—ouch! Instead, sit on the edge of your bed until you can comfortably sit on a ball.

2. Now put one hand on your belly and one hand on your ribs—breathe into your hands—inhale to expand. You should feel your ribs expand and your belly expand away from your spine as the air draws in and fills you up. Sometimes it helps to think about breathing sideways to help bring the air to your ribs. Alternately, visualize inflating a balloon inside your stomach and filling up the balloon with air. Other cues that may be helpful are breathing into your bra strap or opening up an umbrella.

3. Once you have it, focus on the inhale for a few breaths—inhale to expand and feel your ribs inflate, as your belly expands, and bring your awareness to your pelvic floor. Feel space between your sit bones and a sense of fullness in your perineum. Focus just on the in breath for a while and really connect with the feeling of expansion that each inhale brings to your ribs, belly, and pelvic floor.

   The breathing diaphragm moves down as you breathe in and up as you breathe out, and the pelvic floor works in synergy with the diaphragm, so it also descends (expands) as you breathe in and lifts (engages) as you breathe out. The more the diaphragm can move, the more your lungs can expand and the more oxygen you can take in.

4. You've connected with the inhale; now bring your awareness to your exhale. As you breathe out, feel the ribs soften, the belly move inward, and the pelvic floor lift. You may feel less fullness in your perineum, less space between the sit bones, less awareness of the surface of the ball.

5. Once you've connected with the out breath, purse your lips and blow as if you are blowing out birthday candles—it should be a slow audible exhale through pursed lips. How

did that change the sensations? Were you more aware of the movement in your pelvic floor? By pursing your lips, it changes the sensations of pressure and typically heightens the sensation of lift and inward movement of the pelvic floor and belly.

This is the Core Breath—inhale to expand, exhale to engage. Always exhale through pursed lips. And now for the fun part—you will add in some visualizations to really connect with the lifting movement of the pelvic floor as you exhale to engage and voluntarily contract the pelvic.

Imagine as you exhale: preventing a tampon from slipping out, picking up a blueberry with your vagina and anus (not crushing the blueberry, just picking it up!), or lifting your perineum up toward the crown of your head.

Each time you inhale you are relaxing and softening the pelvic floor as it expands. Each time your exhale you are pursing your lips and voluntarily lifting and engaging your pelvic floor as it contracts. Do the Core Breath for 1–3 minutes at least once a day with the other three core exercises.

EXERCISE 2: The Bridge (with Core Breath)

You have probably seen this exercise in the gym or in yoga classes and it is a great exercise on its own but when you add the Core Breath to it, look out mummy tummy! The bridge is also a great glute builder, and great glutes mean a great pelvic floor, and a great pelvic floor means a great inner core!

The cool thing about this exercise is that you are strengthening your glutes *and* giving your babe a gentle hug with your abdominals.

Ensure you have mastered the Core Breath first, as the rest of the exercises add it to movements, and if you don't have good grasp of this foundation exercise then the rest of the exercises will not be as effective.

1. Lie on your back on your yoga mat with your knees bent and feet flat on the floor. Because we want to protect baby, please use a wedge or a stack of pillows under your head, neck, and shoulders.

2. Check for a neutral spine—there should be a gentle curve in your low back with your pubis (pubic bone) in the same line as your pelvis (hip bones).

3. Inhale to expand and then exhale to engage your core.

4. With your core engaged, imagine you have a coin between your butt cheeks and squeeze the coin first before you lift your bum off the floor and before your hamstrings engage. This can be tough at first, especially for runners who have no glutes to begin with or experienced lifters who are hamstring dominant. Keep your neutral spine as you lift and lower.

5. Now inhale to expand as you lower back down.

Repeat this 8–10 times for 1–2 sets daily.

Exercise 3: The Clam

The Clam focuses on the outer glutes—the muscles that will help you hold your leg in side-lying labor and birth positions.

1. Lie on your side with your knees bent and a gentle curve in your low back.

2. Stack your ankles, knees, and hips so you are well aligned.

3. Add in the Core Breath—inhale to expand and then exhale to engage your core.

4. Keeping your heels pressed together, slowly lift the top knee away from the bottom knee.

5. Inhale to expand as you lower the top knee back down.

Repeat 8–10 times for 1–2 sets daily.

Preparing for the Ab Aftermath: Ab Wrapping

Belly binding or wrapping has been performed post-labor and delivery for centuries all over the world, using corsets, wraps, compression garments, and everything in between. The theory is that a woman needs to put everything back in its place as soon as possible during healing, so she can have her figure back ASAP. There is something to be said for encouraging muscles and organs to go back to where they used to be, and it only makes sense that the "sooner the better" approach will help get you there faster. Belly binding helps to create an outer strength while you work on building back some inner strength. It can also be effective beyond the early days postpartum.

But somewhere along the way, here in North America, we have lost the tradition of belly binding. We have moved away from support, maybe because someone, somewhere said that if we support from the outside, we become lazy on the inside. Sure, this can happen. Wearing a support garment postpartum while not doing anything else can create a crutch that might leave you with a flat tummy—while you are wearing the wrap, at least—but a weak core.

The most current research in diastasis shows that any self-healing that will occur will happen in the first 8 weeks postpartum. In other words, if you do nothing, your separation will be the same one year postpartum as it was at eight weeks.

Wrapping your belly during the first 8 weeks not only helps to bring the muscles back together but also allows you to take advantage of this self-healing time. Add a preventive exercise program during pregnancy (like the one in this chapter) and a restorative exercise program postpartum (also in this book). In other words, belly binding must be coupled with proper restorative exercises so you can get out of the wrap and build your own flat tummy from the inside out.

Providing support to the healing connective tissues and muscles, belly wrapping is an age-old tradition that inspired the Bellies Inc. team to design a modern-day version so we moms could reap the benefits without being subjected to the tedious wrapping and being unable to move and breathe. Just like you would wrap the injured tissues and muscles in an ankle strain, so too should you wrap the injured tissues in your abdomen after pregnancy and birth. It is meant to be temporary and done in conjunction with the Core Confidence exercise program.

Just like any product, not all wraps are created equal! Some binders can actually contribute to pelvic floor dysfunction by increasing the intra-abdominal pressure. There are many belly wraps on the market, so research your choice of belly wrap like you would any important product for your health. One option is the version the Bellies Inc. team created called the AB Tank and Wrap, which has light compression in the tank and fully adjustable pelvic, low back, and abdominal support. This offers lift and support with gentle compression rather than tight, top-down cinching that can actually lead to pelvic floor dysfunction.

You'll want to get your belly wrap *before* you have baby so that you can put it on shortly after delivery and take advantage of the most critical healing time for diastasis—the first 8 weeks postpartum. Even if you have a C-section, ab wrapping helps support the cut muscles and can be worn slightly modified to lift the belly away from the incision. I have a link to the high-quality Bellies Inc. AB Tank and Wrap on my website (www.sisinshape.com) under Shop. Consider adding it to your baby shower wish list!

Summary

1. **Perform the Core Confidence exercises daily, or at minimum five times a week.**

    If you are unable to do any of the other exercises in this book due to morning sickness, fatigue, or any of the other challenges that happen during pregnancy, I strongly encourage you to at least do the Core Confidence exercises and go for a 20-minute walk. It may not seem like much, but you are giving your body and baby an amazing gift!

2. **Protect your linea alba: Avoid crunches, planks, or being on all fours and other front-loaded positions at length.**

    Remember, the linea alba is stretched. If you then turn yourself onto all fours for long periods of time, then you will also have the pull of gravity working against your linea alba. Crunches put pressure on the linea alba, round the shoulders, and create downward pressure on the pelvic floor—not what a pregnant mama needs!

3. **Be ready for the ab aftermath: purchase an ab wrap now.**

    The first 8 weeks are the most critical in terms of supporting the connective tissue as it heals and encouraging your abdominal muscles to realign. You'll want to have your ab wrap beforehand so you can put it on in the first days after delivery.

4. **Protect your pelvic floor: Avoid high-impact movements that put on more pressure.**

    This is discussed more at length in chapter 2, yet it's worth repeating here since we are talking in depth about our pelvic floor. Remember how I explained that your pregnant body releases a hormone called relaxin? We don't want to increase your chances of bladder leaks or prolapse, so *Your Fit Pregnancy* programs show you how to stay active and strong (even fit) during your pregnancy without pounding your unstable joints or compromised core. If you have a favorite fitness move, class, or program, just apply your common sense. Are you repeatedly bouncing or putting pressure on your pelvic floor? If so, consider looking for a lower-impact version or activity for the short period of time you are pregnant (and until your pelvic floor is strengthened postpartum to handle the pressure).

Notes: _____

_____

_____

_____

_____

_____

_____

_____

_____

_____

_____

_____

_____

_____

_____

_____

_____

_____

_____

_____

_____

_____

_____

_____

_____

_____

_____

_____

Notes: _____
_____
_____
_____
_____
_____
_____
_____
_____
_____
_____
_____
_____
_____
_____
_____
_____
_____
_____
_____
_____
_____
_____
_____
_____
_____

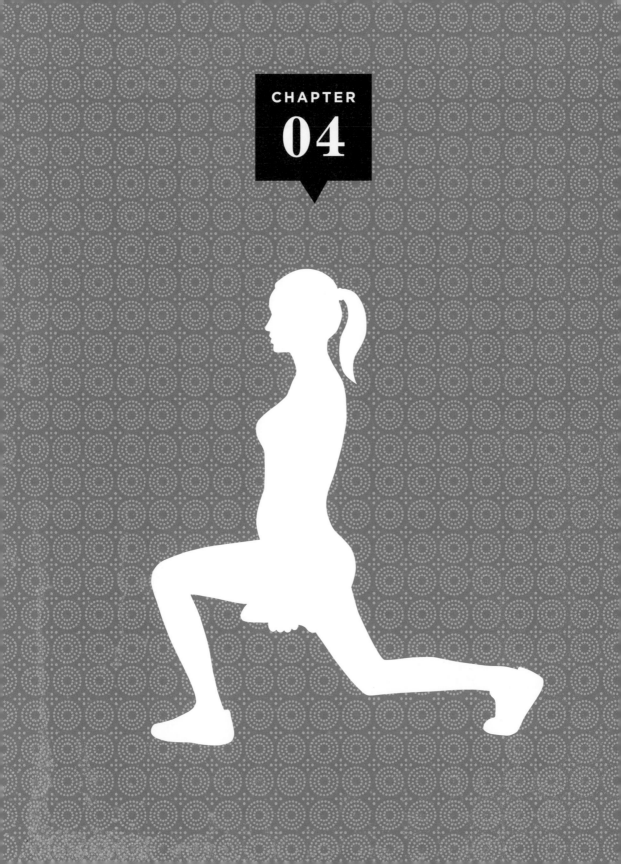

CHAPTER

04

YOUR FIT SECOND TRIMESTER

→ Growing, growing, growing! Trimester two is another step closer to cuddles and kisses but there's lots of work left to do to nurture that little life while nurturing yours!

Your Fit Second Trimester Exercise

My first reaction to most pregnancy fitness routines was how lame they were. The moves were boring, and if you're not into yoga, you're out of luck. Anything that resembled strength moves caused me to yawn just looking at them. There was little variety in even the basic moves, and no progression if you were able to perform more than just a few moves in a session. So how are this book and the routines in it any different?

One of the important aspects of the programs in *Your Fit Pregnancy* is that the strength routines are set up to leverage the power of pace. Increasing your heart rate raises baby's heart rate, and that creates a more mature and stronger cardiovascular system for your baby. We of course don't want to push that little heart rate too high, which means a full-out-heart-racing-out-of-breath pace is too much!

The strength routines in this book are intentionally set up to keep your pace up to get in these amazing cardiovascular benefits while also strengthening your body. A strong body for mommy helps you avoid injuries to susceptible weakened muscles and helps you retain as much lean muscle as possible

throughout your pregnancy. The paced strength training also has rest periods in between sets or circuits not only to allow your muscles to recover before the next set or circuit, but also to allow baby's heart to recover and not be pushed too hard.

You may be curious how *Your Fit Pregnancy* strength training achieves this pace perfection. First of all, it's not the same for each trimester, as it's important that your exercise changes as you are changing! In the first trimester, all of the strength training is set up to use supersets. Supersets are performing two exercises back-to-back before resting. By coupling the exercises, your heart rate is allowed to elevate before you take a rest. In the first trimester program, there are only two exercise performed back-to-back so that you are likely able to lift heavier weights than if you did an entire circuit series of more than two exercises in a row. This way, in your first trimester you may be able to progress in your strength to lay a good foundation for the next two trimesters. At the same time, your pace is benefiting baby's and your cardiovascular system.

Moving on to the second trimester, *Your Fit Pregnancy* puts three or four moves back-to-back before resting. This is done intentionally for two reasons. First, from a pace perspective, you get a naturally elevated heart rate by performing the continuous exercises. The required rest between circuits is there to keep you from pushing it too hard. Second, performing more than just two moves continuously forces you to reduce the weight you are lifting in order to complete all of the repetitions in row. This keeps you and baby safe as you progress in your pregnancy, while maintaining your lean muscle and strength.

In the third trimester, *Your Fit Pregnancy* puts all of your strength exercises into one large continuous circuit. Catching on to why? You'll get amazing pace benefits by continuously moving through each exercise, but still have a forced rest period to make sure your (and baby's) heart rate comes back down before we bring it back up when the circuit is repeated. At the same time, the large circuit-style program leads you to choose lighter weights or just use your body weight as you advance in your pregnancy. While you won't increase your strength or lean muscle development this way, you'll stay safe and do a great job at maintaining what you have in that respect in the last part of your pregnancy.

See how the paced strength training does double if not triple duty? The paced programs with loads of variety in the exercise moves make your exercise more interesting (and less lame). They are also set up to reflect the natural progression of your pregnancy. That's why we call it the power of pace.

How Heavy?

Because we're including regular strength training in your pregnancy fitness, we need to chat about how heavy to lift. Seasoned lifters in particular need to review this section, not just for some new safety adaptations to their lifting but also for some gentle and supportive words about what you may quickly find you can no longer do. It's standard to say that you should be selecting a weight with which you can perform the exercise with excellent form. That is of course true during your pregnancy for strength training. Pelvic floor pressure is of concern if you select too heavy of a weight for a couple reasons:

FIRST, while weight training is low impact, some exercises, especially standing lower body moves, will put pressure on your pelvic floor. These are the ones we want to be most careful with for the same reasons I gave for high-impact exercise like running. The relaxin hormone relaxes everything, and repeatedly or forcefully pressing down on your relaxed pelvic floor could have long-term negative effects. For this reason, I've specifically chosen many of the strength training moves to be done while seated, especially in the latter part of your pregnancy, as the weight of the baby puts pressure on your pelvic floor. There is no need to add more pressure with heavily weighted moves.

SECOND, when a too-heavy weight is selected, most people force out their breath while they strain to complete the repetition. See for yourself: Give a little grunt or push out your breath. Notice where some pressure goes to? Yup, that's right, to your lower core and pelvic floor: exactly where we don't want unnecessary pressure.

So, how heavy? Common sense tells us not to pick up the 100-pound dumbbells with baby on board, but ensure that you become aware that if at any point you are feeling as if you are bearing down on your pelvic floor to complete the move, it's too heavy. On the flip side, if you feel disengaged while completing the move because it is so easy, then you can probably select a heavier weight in order to reap the many benefits of strength training. It comes down to self-awareness, of course, of excellent form but also of the breath you are using to execute the exercise and/or where you are feeling the exertion.

For the experienced lifters reading this book: Hi!—fist pump—bicep flex. I also considered myself an advanced lifter coming into my pregnancy, and so I thought all of the "take it slower" advice was part of the lame stuff people who are not into fitness say. Therefore, I thought that advice didn't apply to me. I was served humble pie quickly around week 7 as my body struggled to complete lifts that had been easy to me pre-pregnancy and my instincts told me to pull back. After I dove into all of the research on pelvic floor health and pregnancy fitness, I'm grateful I listened to my instincts, but in the interim, I struggled with accepting not being able to push it during my workouts. I will forever be grateful for the advice my close (and very fit) friend Meaghan told me over lunch around 16 weeks (see Meaghan's Preggo Pal Profile in chapter 1). Meaghan is a stunning fit mom of two, so if she had said she rubbed mayonnaise on her tummy to get her abs like that post-baby I probably would have! Anyway, Meaghan gently told me how much she struggled with her level of fitness during her pregnancy. She was sick and exhausted, and despite her top level of fitness coming into pregnancy, doing the same type of workouts or even maintaining her fitness was not going to happen. But she knew the importance of exercising for herself and baby, so she did her best. Her best was 20 minutes each day of walking on her treadmill. Looking at that beautiful fit mom, proof of the advice, I finally accepted that pulling back was okay. If you don't have a friend like that in your life, let me be that person for you. Do your best for you and baby, but don't get down on yourself for having to pull back on your choice of weights or reducing the length of your sessions. After your body is retrained postpartum, you'll get back at it like the awesome fitness freak you are!

Pre- and Post-Workout Nutrition

The intensity level of *Your Fit Pregnancy* programs do not require specialized pre- or post-workout nutrition. The basic nutrition guidelines in previous chapters will cover you just fine, because it is much more important for you to focus on your overall daily nutrition than to fuss around with what to eat when. While I try to reassure my lifestyle fitness clients about this fact, they still look for these pre- and post-workout guidelines, so here they are!

Aim to eat a meal that includes a carbohydrate and protein every 2–3 hours. If you're eating in this time range, then there is no need for a pre-workout meal or snack.

If it's been more than 3 hours since your last meal, have a small snack 30–60 minutes before your workout that includes a protein and a carbohydrate. An example would be a cup of low-fat Greek yogurt with some berries or at least part of a grilled chicken sandwich on whole wheat bread.

Post-workout, especially on strength training days, aim to eat a good source of protein and carbohydrate within 30 minutes after your workout. From my more intense training days, I continued my habit of having a high-quality post-workout whey-based protein shake that included a carbohydrate like a banana. Greek yogurt or a chicken sandwich are also good post-workout options given the low level of intensity in *Your Fit Pregnancy* workouts.

"Water helps curb fatigue, curbs appetite, as your body can confuse insufficient hydration with hunger. Water also helps with the digestion and tummy troubles that are prevalent during pregnancy."

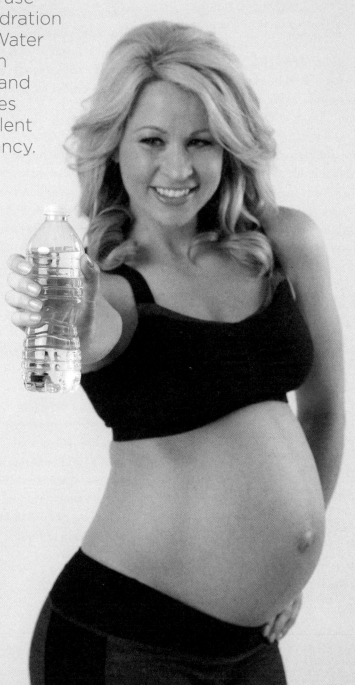

Water!

Everyone knows to drink lots of water, but the issue here isn't knowledge but execution. Water is one of the three fundamentals of *Your Fit Pregnancy* nutrition (see page 12). Water is basic yet critical to keeping everything functioning well in your (and baby's) body. Water also helps curb fatigue as well as appetite, as your body can confuse insufficient hydration with hunger. Drinking enough water also helps with the digestion and tummy troubles that are prevalent during pregnancy. You may be wary of water if you feel you are retaining it; however, drinking enough water actually helps with swelling because more water helps flush out extra fluid.

In my initial intake call with a new client, I ask about water consumption. The majority of them quickly respond, "Oh, yes, I drink lots of water!" I then ask them to explain the volume of their water bottle they most often drink out of and how many times they fill it up. Based on their response we do a little math. Too often I uncover that they are not drinking as much as they thought and not nearly enough to meet their daily drinking quota.

So how much is enough, and is it different for an active pregnant woman?

At minimum, a pregnant woman should be drinking at least 2 liters (approximately 64 ounces) of water a day. Since you are active you should be aiming for 3 liters each day. The easiest way to get your water in is to use a large refillable water bottle and know how many of those bottles you need to drink to make it to your water quota. If you're drinking less than 2 liters a day now, gradually add more water into your day so that your body becomes adjusted to the increase in water and you can avoid having to pee every 2 minutes (instead of the every 10 minutes it seems you are going these days!).

A frequently asked question is "Do you count other liquids that you are drinking in your water quota?" Most literature says yes, you can include fruit juices, noncaffeinated beverages, and watery types of fruits or vegetables in your daily drinking count. However, I strongly encourage you to get used to drinking plain simple water and count only that for getting in your 2–3 liters a day. Also, do you need to drink plain water? It's tempting to flavor your water for taste, as plain water has, well, no taste. However, you will get used to drinking plain water after a couple weeks, and I strongly encourage you to drink plain simple water or adding only a squeeze of natural lemon to flavor it. Too many flavor tricks add unnecessary sugars and sweeteners into your diet. Spice up your food and eat fruit, but when it comes to water, drink the plain simple stuff!

Calories: Can I Eat More Now?

In the first trimester we chatted about not needing to add more calories unless your doctor advised you to do so. So can you eat more now? How's this for an answer: Probably, but just a bit, and likely not as much as you think.

A healthy-weight pregnant woman needs to add only 250–300 calories a day to build her baby in the second and third trimesters. That's actually not much extra food. To put it in perspective, that would be *one* of the following extras in your daily eating:

- 1 medium apple and 12 almonds
- A small glass of milk and a piece of plain whole wheat toast
- 3 spoonfuls of peanut butter (yup, just 3!)

Get the idea? That's one additional small snack, and that's it! How disappointing, right? Eating more than what baby needs to grow means *you* are eating more than you need,

and excess calories mean extra weight gain. Think that's not a big deal? Yes, I agree, a few extra pounds isn't a big deal. I admit I had at least 5–7 of those pounds stuck to my backside at the end of my pregnancy, but the truth is that weight loss is never easy. Unsurprisingly, losing weight after baby (whether it's 8 weeks after or 80 weeks after) is not any more fun or easier. Also, a host of health issues for you and baby comes with being overweight! So while you want to ensure that you are getting lots of nourishment for you and baby, use the Handy Portion Sizes guide on page 35 to keep unnecessary weight gain in check and your nutrition balanced.

Micronutrients: Little Powerhouses

We've chatted about *macro*nutrients (proteins, carbs, and fats), and you'll recall that those are the nutrients we needs in large quantities. Now let's take our basic nutrition knowledge one step further and look at *micro*nutrients as the third pillar of *Your Fit Pregnancy* nutrition.

The term *micro* means "small," and you'll remember *nutrients* means "a substance that provides nourishment essential for growth and maintenance of life." Put those together and *micronutrients* means what you need in small quantities to nourish and grow life. These are the vitamins and minerals you need, even if only in small amounts, that play an important role in baby development and your well-being. A lack of micronutrients can lead to stunted growth or increased risk of various diseases. Little powerhouses indeed!

I found learning about all the micronutrients a bit overwhelming. Vitamins A, B, C, D, K, and it seems they go on and on until triple ZZZ! Then you have minerals: calcium, iron, potassium, and I think there's gold, myrrh, and frankincense? Okay, you get the idea. There are a lot of them, and while they are super important, I don't want you to get bogged down in the details so that you forget the basics of where they come from and how to get them.

The secret is nutrient-dense food. *Nutrient-dense* is another technical term that is thrown around a lot these days. Simply put, it means that the ratio that compares the amount of calories the food gives you to the amount of nutrients contained in the food. Low-calorie foods with many nutrients (like fruits and vegetables) have higher nutrient densities. To ensure that you are getting in your important micronutrients, you don't

need to know that tomatoes are a source of vitamin A, C, K, potassium, and folate. That knowledge doesn't help you get a healthy baby. What does? Filling your plate with a variety of nutrient-dense foods (fruits, vegetables, whole grains, lean proteins, and healthy fats).

By making good choices with your macronutrients you likely are making good choices with your micronutrients. Sneaking in extra veggies helps a lot, because while they do not hold a significant macronutrient count compared to most foods (two large handfuls of spinach contains less than 2 grams of carbs), they pack a powerful micronutrient punch!

Revisit the Handy Portion Sizes guide and look at it differently. Instead of seeing macronutrients, see all the incredible micronutrient powerhouses!

This is often where clients ask if they can take a vitamin and/or mineral pill to cover their micronutrient needs. Even though we feel we are advanced as a society in the area of food science, we actually know very little about the complex nutrient values of our food. Over the decades, scientists have attempted to break down, isolate, and recreate the properties of our food. Yet there continue to be new discoveries (daily, it seems) about the amazing properties of our food. As a result, I strongly encourage clients to choose as many nutrient-dense foods as possible and then supplement with high-quality vitamins and minerals in consultation with their doctor.

Preggo Power Foods Meal Planner and Sample Menu: Second Trimester

Packing a micronutrient punch in each of the Preggo Power recipes gets all the good stuff into your daily diet while still tasting amazing.

Breakfast

CHOOSE ONE OF:

- Easy Italian Baked Eggs
- Coconut Flour Apple Pancakes
- Pumpkin Granola Yogurt Parfait
- Protein smoothie that has all macronutrients (look for a high-quality meal replacement type of protein shake or add in fats and carbohydrates such as almond butter and a banana).

Snack Mid-Morning and Late Afternoon

CHOOSE ONE FOR EACH MID-MORNING AND LATE AFTERNOON SNACK:

- Peach Cobbler Greek Yogurt
- Easy Egg Muffins
- Hardboiled egg and an apple
- 24 almonds (1.5–2 servings of nuts) and a serving of fruit

Lunch & Dinner

ANY OF THE PREGGO POWER LUNCH/DINNER RECIPES *PLUS* 1 SERVING OF COMPLEX CARBOHYDRATES (WHOLE WHEAT BREAD, BROWN RICE, ETC.).

- Build a meal that is well balanced with sources of protein, carbohydrates, and fats. Load up on veggies for an extra power boost.

Evening Snack

CHOOSE ONE OF:

- 1-Minute Banana Split Mug Cake
- Fig and Chocolate Frozen Protein Fudge
- Mint Chocolate Green Protein Smoothie
- Glass of low-fat milk and a piece of whole wheat toast with natural peanut butter
- Veggies and 1/3 cup of hummus

On a Sunday morning, bake up the Easy Italian Baked Eggs, as they sneak in loads of vitamins and minerals in the tomato sauce, spinach, and whole eggs. Or try the Coconut Flour Apple Pancakes, which are a good source of vitamin B as well as iron and potassium.

Each snack is bursting with micronutrients (and flavor!) in peaches, spinach, bananas, and more!

The rest of the snacks and meals are well balanced with their macronutrients and were selected to be packed with baby-building nutrients.

As we're eating a bit more for our second trimester of baby building, enjoy a nutrient-packed evening dessert—so yummy you won't believe you're nourishing baby with your treat!

Your Fit Second Trimester Workouts

I want you to be as prepared as possible for the upcoming third trimester, in which belly size and weight as well as stability limitations take over. Therefore, the focus in your second trimester will be on maintaining strength and flexibility.

Of course we can't ignore that growing belly! These exercises have been selected and modified to be comfortable yet effective for you and your bump. Each workout will take you approximately 30 minutes to complete.

In your second trimester, keep these habits in your exercise:

Incorporate at least three Core Confidence moves each day (refer to chapter 3).

Go for an additional 20- to 30-minute walk or low-impact cardio activity if your schedule permits.

YOUR FIT SECOND TRIMESTER						
Day 1	Day 2	Day 3	Day 4	Day 5	Day 6	Day 7
Strength Train: full body	Cardio Activity	Strength Train: upper body	Strength Train: lower body	Yoga / Stretch	Strength Train: full body	Cardio Activity
Include at least three Core Confidence moves each day (chapter 3).						
If your schedule permits, add 20–30 minutes of walking or low-impact cardio activity.						

STRENGTH TRAINING

The Basics:

For each exercise, choose a weight that ensures you are not straining or compromising your form at any point during the exercise.

Keep progressing! If you could easily perform five more repetitions, consider increasing the weight for the next set.

Rest between circuits. Take adequate rest in between each circuit set to ensure that you could easily carry on a normal conversation while exercising. This may be as little as 30 seconds or up to a couple minutes of rest.

This program's exercises are to be completed as two different circuits per workout. This means that you will complete all exercises in the first circuit (circuit A) for the prescribed number of reps, rest, and then repeat the moves in that circuit. You continue this format until you've reached your target number of sets, then you move on to the second circuit (circuit B).

This circuit style of workout will naturally force you to decrease the amount of weight that you are lifting in each exercise compared to the workouts in the first trimester. This is for the safety of both you and baby.

Stop exercising if you feel you are pushing it. Some days are like that— always listen to your body.

BEGINNER: Complete 1–2 sets of each exercise for 12–15 repetitions. Choose a light weight or use your own body weight. For exercises that indicate the use of a barbell, you may substitute a resistance band with handles to perform the movement.

Finish your workout with a 15-minute walk.

DAY 1—STRENGTH TRAIN: FULL BODY					
CIRCUIT A			CIRCUIT B		
A1	A2	A3	B1	B2	B3
Walking lunges	Front raise with dumbbells	Incline chest flye	Squat*	Side lateral raise	Barbell curl

*Only if you have excellent form. Keep weight light to avoid straining or pushing through the pelvic area.

DAY 3—STRENGTH TRAIN: UPPER BODY

CIRCUIT A				CIRCUIT B		
A1	A2	A3	A4	B1	B2	B3
Wide-grip lat pull-down	Seated shoulder press	Incline chest press	Bent-over standing row	Rear delt flye (standing wide legged)	Concentration curl	Dumbbell punches

DAY 4—STRENGTH TRAIN: LOWER BODY

CIRCUIT A			CIRCUIT B		
A1	A2	A3	B1	B2	B3
Leg extensions (toes straight)	Leg extensions (toes out)	Standing kickback on cable machine	Squat*	Bird dog	Calf raises (toes: 1 set in, 1 set out, 1 set straight)

*Only if you have excellent form. Keep weight light to avoid straining or pushing through the pelvic area.

DAY 6—STRENGTH TRAIN: FULL BODY

CIRCUIT A			CIRCUIT B		
A1	A2	A3	B1	B2	B3
Goblet sumo squat	Tricep rope extension	Preggo push-up	**BEGINNER:** Front lunge	Side lateral raises	Overhead tricep extension (one-arm)
			INT/ADV: Cable pull-through*		

*Alternate exercise is a seated hamstring curl. This machine is found at most gyms and is a great alternative for working the backs of your legs.

" Rock Your Tiger Stripes "

MY WHOLE LIFE I was somewhat fit, but just going through the motions in the gym and not taking my nutrition seriously. I mean, I went to the gym and lifted and even taught aerobics. Why couldn't I enjoy my candy bars, chips, and sodas every day and get the results I really wanted? I truly thought I could have my cake and eat it, too.

My eyes were opened when I got pregnant with our first child. I was sick most of the pregnancy, in and out of the hospital, and on bed rest at 28 weeks (for preterm labor) until my C-section at 38 weeks. Let me tell you what happens with the mind-set I had before. Oh, that whole "you can enjoy your junk food and still be fit" doesn't really work when you are sick or on bed rest and aren't exercising. Needless to say, this mama gained 70 pounds and was in total shock once I came home from the hospital from a C-section, took a look in the mirror, and realized, *Oh crap. My hips, butt, legs, and arms didn't go down once the baby came out*. I mean, I knew it wouldn't be that miraculous, but a girl can dream, right?

I was dealing with some severe postpartum depression, and although I loved my child, the weight gain was taking a toll on me emotionally. I thought I would never be the same again. I sat down on the floor one day and cried—sobbed, really. I realized I needed to stop feeling sorry for myself, get off my butt, and *fight for it*. Right then I decided to start hitting the gym. The only time I could go was before work, so I would go at 6 a.m. while my husband would be home with our son.

Remember, before pregnancy I was fit, so it was humbling stepping foot into the gym at that weight. I was so much larger and I had nothing to wear. I remember going in a big, frumpy T-shirt

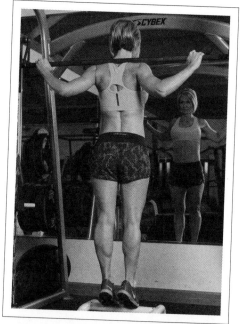

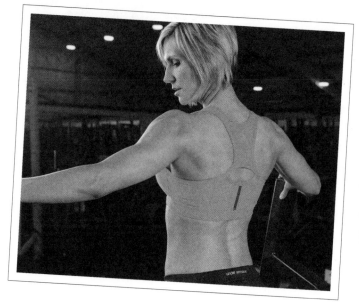

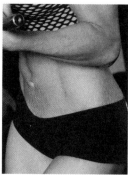

and my husband's shorts. Once I started to see results, it motivated me to work out even harder. It took a full year, but by my son's first birthday I felt healthy and fit again.

Fast-forward three and a half years. I found myself pregnant again, and history repeated itself. I couldn't believe my body would balloon out that big again! I wasn't on bed rest, I didn't eat complete junk, and I still gained around 70 pounds. I had another C-section, and when I could get back to working out, I did. This time we had installed a gym in our garage, but working out at home takes discipline, and I knew I had a lot of work to do. *No* excuses. *No* giving up. I did it, and I'm in the best shape of my life now after having two children. I will also tell you that these two huge pregnancies came with some serious "tiger stripes," but I rock them the best way I can!

Never give up, do the work, and be proud of your body (we grew tiny humans in there!). For me, those stretch marks are a daily reminder of my journey and how far I have come. Rock those bodies, ladies, tiger stripes and all. Create your own story, get your "after" picture, and go inspire!

> ▶ You can connect with Dani at danigeturgunz.com as she inspires women to be their best. Just a note, flexing your "gunz" is a requirement!

INTERMEDIATE: Complete 2-3 sets of each exercise for 12-15 repetitions.

If performing 2 sets, then finish your workout with a 15-minute walk.

ADVANCED: Complete 3-4 sets of each exercise for 10-12 repetitions. The repetitions are fewer than for the intermediate level as it is assumed that you are choosing a more challenging weight yet still executing the moves with excellent form.

CARDIO

The Basics:

Choose a low-impact activity that raises your heart rate slightly for 20-30 minutes, ensuring that you could easily carry on a normal conversation while exercising.

The activity does not need to be performed for a continuous 30 minutes. Two 15-minute sessions are equally as effective.

Remember that you are getting in cardiovascular benefits for you and baby during your strength training sessions, too!

Activity options for days 2 and 7:
- Walking
- Elliptical machine
- Stepper machine
- Swimming
- Stationary bike

YOGA

This yoga-based sequence of five prenatal stretches and restorative poses takes you from standing to sitting to lying down.

Hold or gently move through each pose for 2-3 minutes, focusing on your breath.

Breathe slowly in and out through your nose.

Gently move your body through the full ranges of motion, never straining during a pose.

Repeat the sequence for a total of two sequences.

DAY 5—YOGA / STRETCH				
1	2	3	4	5
Standing quad stretch supported by wall	Cat/Cow	Runner's lunge with block	Seated straddle with chest twist	Side-lying pose supported with pillows

MY FIT BUMP

SECOND TRIMESTER (16 WEEKS)

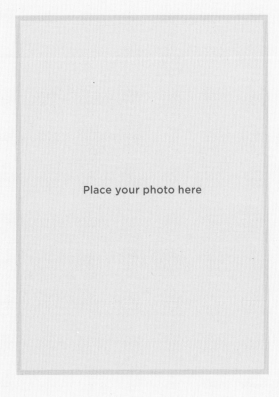

Place your photo here

MY FIT BUMP

SECOND TRIMESTER (20 WEEKS)

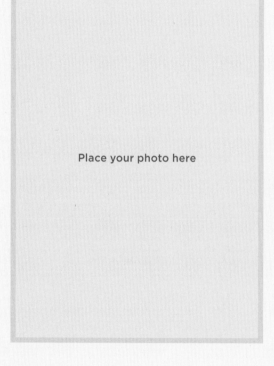

Place your photo here

MY FIT BUMP

SECOND TRIMESTER (24 WEEKS)

Place your photo here

THEN . . . AND NOW

PRE-BABY	BABY ON BOARD

My fav exercise was _____

_____

_____

_____

My fav exercise is _____

_____

_____

_____

My workout clothes were_____

_____

_____

_____

My workout clothes are _____

_____

_____

_____

My fav healthy food was_____

_____

_____

_____

My fav healthy food is_____

_____

_____

_____

My fav junk food was _____

_____

_____

_____

My fav junk food is _____

_____

_____

_____

I was strong at_____

_____

_____

_____

I am strong at _____

_____

_____

_____

MY FIT SECOND TRIMESTER | NUTRITION

MY TYPICAL DAILY MENU

Breakfast _____
_____

❑ Water

Mid-morning _____
_____

❑ Water

Lunch _____
_____

❑ Water

Mid-afternoon _____
_____

❑ Water

Dinner _____
_____

❑ Water

Evening (optional) _____
_____

❑ Water

MY FIT SECOND TRIMESTER | NUTRITION
SHOPPING LIST

Lean Proteins
- ❏ _____
- ❏ _____
- ❏ _____
- ❏ _____

Complex Carbs
- ❏ _____
- ❏ _____
- ❏ _____
- ❏ _____

Fruits & Veggies
- ❏ _____
- ❏ _____
- ❏ _____
- ❏ _____

Healthy Fats
- ❏ _____
- ❏ _____
- ❏ _____
- ❏ _____

MY FIT SECOND TRIMESTER

EXERCISE & TRACKING SHEET

EXERCISE NAME	MONTH 4 (REPS & LBS)	MONTH 5 (REPS & LBS)	MONTH 6 (REPS & LBS)

CORE CONFIDENCE TRACKER:

Put a checkmark below each time you strengthen your core & pelvic floor.

❑ ❑ ❑ ❑ ❑ ❑ ❑ ❑ ❑ ❑ ❑ ❑

CARDIO

Note your cardio activity this trimester:

_____

_____

_____

MY FIT SECOND TRIMESTER

EXERCISE & TRACKING SHEET

EXERCISE NAME	MONTH 4 (REPS & LBS)	MONTH 5 (REPS & LBS)	MONTH 6 (REPS & LBS)

CORE CONFIDENCE TRACKER:

Put a checkmark below each time you strengthen your core & pelvic floor.

❑ ❑ ❑ ❑ ❑ ❑ ❑ ❑ ❑ ❑ ❑ ❑

CARDIO

Note your cardio activity this trimester:

_____

_____

MY FIT SECOND TRIMESTER

EXERCISE & TRACKING SHEET

EXERCISE NAME	MONTH 4 (REPS & LBS)	MONTH 5 (REPS & LBS)	MONTH 6 (REPS & LBS)

CORE CONFIDENCE TRACKER:

Put a checkmark below each time you strengthen your core & pelvic floor.

❑ ❑ ❑ ❑ ❑ ❑ ❑ ❑ ❑ ❑ ❑ ❑

CARDIO

Note your cardio activity this trimester:

_____

_____

_____

CHAPTER

05

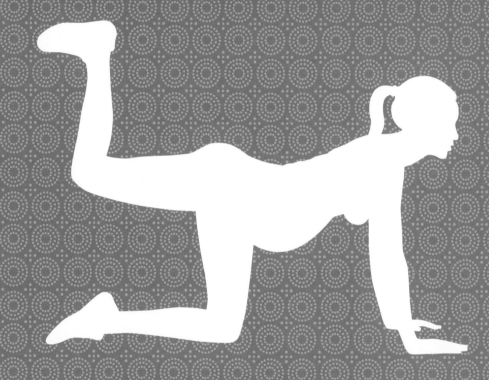

YOUR FIT THIRD TRIMESTER

→ The home stretch is here. With a whole new life is just around the corner, let's finish strong!

Your Fit Third Trimester Exercise

Exercising gets particularly interesting when you can't see your toes anymore. Many of the fitness moves you may be familiar with simply won't work at this stage due to the size of your belly! This is where we reach deep into our exercise library and pull out the moves that are effective yet still doable with your sizable bump. *Your Fit Pregnancy* exercises in the last trimester leverage the following:

Seated moves. Take the pressure off your pelvic floor and keep yourself stable. For example, a seated overhead press is just as effective for your shoulders as a standing overhead press; however, your core and low back are more effectively stabilized while seated. The seated exercise machines at the gym are also great for isolating a muscle, as well as easy weight selection with a pin or dial. Seated leg extensions and seated hamstring curls became regular moves in my last trimester to keep my legs strong and baby safe!

Cable machine. This underutilized resistance-training machine has an infinite number of ways to use it if you know how. The bonus of the cable machine in your third trimester is that you can adjust how far you stand from the weight stack to accommodate your bump! You can also easily adjust the pin on the weight stack to move the weight up or down without hauling around dumbbells. As I progressed in my third trimester the pin on the weight stack was set lighter and lighter, and yet the movement and muscles targeted were able to remain the same.

Body weight moves. Now that your tummy is getting heavier (and heavier!) by the day, I encourage you to not only lighten up the weights you choose but also use just your body weight, especially for lower body moves. Your own body weight is providing ample resistance for a squat or lunge at this stage!

Dirty Looks at the Gym

During my first pregnancy, I vividly recall being at the gym the week I was due. I walked (waddled) to the weight rack and selected a light set of dumbbells, seated myself, and did some overhead shoulder presses. As I was returning the weights to the rack, I passed another gym-goer who looked at me with disgust and shook his head. I was taken aback so much by his reaction that I cut my workout short. As much as I tried, I couldn't get his look out of my mind.

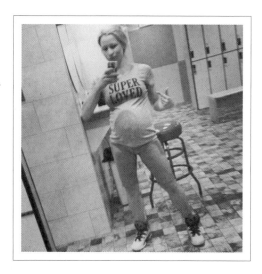

Fast-forward four years later to my second pregnancy, and I was even more regular at the gym. I would go to the gym close to my office on my lunch break. I would do my 4–6 strength exercises and a bit of light cardio or swimming. On days when I was a tired, I went into the studio to do some breathing and a few prenatal yoga poses. My gym visits were at the same time every day, and so the regular lunchtime crowd became familiar with my presence and growing bump. As my pregnancy progressed, I half expected to get a dirty look from another gym-goer. Yet this time it was different. Most days I got a thumbs-up or an encouraging comment. Folks would talk about their kids and how they (or their wives) stayed active during their pregnancy (while everyone who hadn't said they wished they had). No one talked to me during my first pregnancy at the gym. So what was different?

I was caught off guard by the dirty look in my first pregnancy; however, in pregnancy number 2, that experience helped me to accept that it could happen again. Yet for baby, and myself, I confidently chose to be active anyway. In being prepared for the possibility of a dirty look, I actually wore a bigger smile and held my head a bit higher during my workouts. I regularly wore a big T-shirt that said "Super Loved" and high-top pink running shoes. The entire world seems to feel the obligation to pass judgment on you, as a pregnant woman, and give you advice. It's as if your belly wears a sign that says OPEN FOR YOUR OPINION! Yes, it's pretty cool to get a thumbs-up, but dirty looks can hurt your hormonally charged feelings. The reality is that you cannot control others' reactions to you, but you can control how you react. Why not slap on a smile and a pair of pink high-tops to meet those reactions?

"I'll Get in Shape after Baby"

We are into the final stretch, and being active is becoming a lot harder! You're getting bigger (and bigger) and you may feel really (really) tired. Ugh. That motivation you started out with is lagging and aspirations of "being fit" might be switching to "I'll just get in shape after baby." Before you hang up your sneakers until you're pushing a baby stroller, consider the following three points:

1. Why did you decide to include fitness during your pregnancy when you began? When my clients' motivation is starting to lag, I often pull out the personal "why" that they wrote out when we started on their fitness journey. As the days, weeks, and even months slip by, we easily drift away from our core

"why" as life distracts us and, well, continues to happen.

Your "why" likely includes benefits to you and baby, such as boosting baby's brain maturity, keeping your blood pressure in check, and reducing the risk of many health issues. However, do not allow your "why" to become a "should"—a should is not powerful enough to keep you motivated. You "should" do a lot of things, including making your bed, but it's the deeper "whys" that spur us to act even on days we don't feel like it.

2. It doesn't get easier. The saying "A good plan now is better than a perfect plan tomorrow" is sound advice when you're thinking you'll just get in shape after baby instead of doing your best to stay active now. The birthing process takes an immense toll on your body, and you may recover even more slowly after birth than you anticipate. Being prepared now is the only thing you can control, especially since recovering from childbirth is no joke. It's not the "six weeks and you're clear" that too many believe. Interrupted sleep and juggling a new (or bigger) family only adds to the challenges of getting back in shape.

3. Take the pressure of being fit off.

In the final weeks of my pregnancy you'd see me paddling around in the pool, looking more like a whale than a fish and doing some halfhearted lunges or body weight squats. I didn't impress anyone with my fitness feats, and yet as I progressed in my pregnancy it became clearer that this wasn't about being fit—*Your Fit Pregnancy* is about moving. Moving to keep our muscles awake. Moving to make our joined hearts beat a bit quicker. Moving to breathe in new oxygen. Take off any pressure you've put on yourself to being fit and shift your focus to moving, most days, just a bit.

Your Fit Third Trimester Nutrition

The final stretch can be the one filled with the most temptation. Your commitment to making healthy choices may start to wane as baby is almost here. Don't throw in the towel (or baby blanket) yet! There is a whole new set of tricks you can pull out to make better choices for you and baby.

Cravings

Pickles and ice cream—please! There are few hotter topics among pregnant women than what cravings they are having. In my first pregnancy, I too often sent my husband out at all hours of the evening to fetch that important must-have food. Guilty!

Fortunately, in pregnancy number 2, I discovered that there are many ways to deal with these cravings in a way that actually nourish you and baby. Yes, even when the craving is for ice cream! The secret was in teaming up with genius Registered Holistic Nutritionist Christal Sczebel (aka Nutritionist in the Kitch). Christal has a knack for creating indulgent, easy-to-make recipes that still pack a powerful nutrition punch! I've shared my favorite craving-squashing recipes created by Christal in this book, but for more recipes check out Christal's website www.nutritionistinthekitch.com.

Next time a craving hits, don't send your hubby packing—instead try one of these Preggo Power recipes!

SWEET CRAVING?
- Peach Cobbler Greek Yogurt
- Fig and Chocolate Frozen Protein Fudge
- Healthy Crustless Meyer Lemon Cheesecake with Berry "Compote"
- 1-Minute Banana Split Mug Cake

SALTY CRAVING?

- Hummus and Kale Deviled Eggs
- Sweet + Salty Slow Cooker Cashew Chicken
- Easy Slow Cooker Pulled Chicken
- 20-Minute Chicken Tortilla Soup
- Grilled or Baked Mini Tropical Chicken Pizza
- Veggies and hummus

ICE CREAM!?

- Mint Chocolate Green Protein Smoothie
- Orange "Creamsicle" Smoothie
- Healthy Almond Pistachio Frozen Yogurt
- Strawberries and "Cream" Chocolate Chunk Protein "Ice Cream"

There's No Room!

Feeling stuffed full of baby these days? As baby grows, she is taking more real estate in your tummy, and eating to nourish her and you is becoming a challenge. This increases the importance of choosing those nutrient-dense foods we talked about in trimester 2 as often as you can to ensure you and baby are getting those power vitamins and minerals. However, it's the volume eating that poses a problem. A big salad doesn't seem possible to fit in there alongside baby. So how do you fit in good nutrition?

SNACKING AND MINI-MEALS. Snacking often and having mini-meals become important tools in your nutrition in the final trimester. Take any meal and split it in half and eat every couple hours. It seemed I was always snacking on a few spoonfuls of something at my desk in the last trimester! If your day is mostly on the go, choose portable snacks like apples, almonds, and low-fat string cheese. Invest in a nice lunch bag so that you can take your healthy food with you. No one will judge the pregnant lady digging her spoon into a yogurt!

SMOOTHIES. Drinking your nutrients allows you to pack in a bunch of nutrient volume without having to munch on mouthfuls of food. I blended spinach, cooked sweet potatoes, flaxseed, fruit, and almond milk into my smoothies. Buying a quality shaker bottle allows you to blend your smoothie at home, then take it with you for a mid-morning snack or just to sip on while you go through your day.

Takeout and Eating Out

In your last trimester, after a long day of work you may find yourself struggling with cooking dinner every night. Getting takeout and eating out become very appealing meal options. You can make good choices for you and baby while eating away from your kitchen; however, there are a few key tips to keep in mind.

LOOK FOR QUALITY MACROS AND MICROS. Since we're now familiar with both macro and micronutrients, let's take a look at your favorite takeout food from this perspective. Pizza, for example, is dough, tomato sauce, cheese, and toppings. The dough is a dense carbohydrate and cheese is a high fat source with only a touch of protein. Toppings of pepperoni or bacon are fatty sources of protein. There are few micronutrient high points with this takeout. So what did you and your baby get with the pizza? A whole lot of carbs and fat, but few micronutrients and not much protein. This is not to say "don't eat pizza"— on the contrary, I love pizza! But to make up for the pizza's nutritional low points, pair your one or two slices of takeout pizza with a nice green salad drizzled with a bit of lemon juice. Have a protein ice cream for dessert, like the Strawberries and "Cream" Chocolate Chunk "Ice Cream" on page 193, or ensure you are getting sufficient protein in the rest of your day.

WHAT ABOUT "HEALTHY" OPTIONS IN RESTAURANTS? Too often "healthy"-sounding options are worse for you than the burger and fries. Veggies, a lean protein, and a complex carb would be an ideal option. However, the only way to know if the "healthy" option is actually healthy is to look at the restaurant's nutrition stats ahead of time. Salads are often packed with cheese, dried fruit, nuts, and fat- and sugar-laden dressings. When ordering, ask for anything fatty or sugary on the side so you can control how much you put on. In particular, for dressing ask for just olive oil and vinegar, as restaurant dressings taste amazing because of their sizable fat and sugar content.

HANDY PORTIONS STILL APPLY. Restaurant portion sizes are often two or three times larger then the sensible portions shown in the Handy Portion Sizes guide on page 35. The cool thing about those swollen hands of yours is that they still go with you to restaurants! So take them out when eyeballing your plate. Use any leftovers for an easy lunch or dinner the next day.

Preggo Power Foods Meal Planner and Sample Menu: Third Trimester

Cravings and a stuffed tummy may make you lose your appetite for healthy eating. However, with recipes this delicious your cravings will be satisfied and your taste buds watering to get your fill of nutritious food.

And remember we're eating just a bit more for our third trimester baby building, so enjoy a nutrient-packed evening "treat"!

Breakfast

CHOOSE ONE OF:

- Any of the Preggo Power breakfast recipes, like Chunky Monkey Oatmeal
- Protein smoothie that has all macro-nutrients (look for a high-quality meal replacement protein shake or add in fats and carbohydrates such as almond butter and a banana).

Snack Mid-Morning and Late Afternoon

FOR BOTH MID-MORNING AND LATE AFTERNOON CHOOSE ONE OF:

- Strawberry Kiwi Chia Greek Yogurt
- Tuna Tomato Bites
- Hardboiled egg and an apple
- 24 almonds (1.5–2 servings of nuts) and a serving of fruit

Lunch & Dinner

ANY OF THE PREGGO POWER LUNCH/DINNER RECIPES PLUS 1 SERVING OF COMPLEX CARBOHYDRATES (WHOLE WHEAT BREAD, BROWN RICE, ETC.). EACH RECIPE IS PACKED WITH BABY-BUILDING NUTRIENTS.

- Build a meal that is well balanced with sources of protein, carbohydrates, and fats. Load up on veggies for an extra power boost.

Evening Snack

CHOOSE ONE OF:

- Healthy Almond Pistachio Frozen Yogurt
- Hummus and Kale Deviled Eggs
- Healthy Crustless Meyer Lemon Cheesecake with Berry "Compote"
- Glass of low-fat milk and a piece of whole wheat toast with natural peanut butter
- Veggies and 1/3 cup of hummus

Your Fit Third Trimester Workouts

That baby bump is no longer just a little speed bump. As your third trimester progresses, get ready to feel *huge*! Exercise becomes more challenging, as you need to navigate your exercise moves to make room for a front-seat passenger. These exercises have been specifically selected and modified to be comfortable yet effective for you and your bump. Each workout will take you approximately 20–30 minutes to complete.

In your third trimester, keep these habits in your exercise:

Incorporate at least three Core Confidence moves each day (refer to chapter 3).

Go for an additional 20- to 30-minute walk or low-impact cardio activity if your schedule permits.

STRENGTH TRAINING

The Basics:

For each exercise, choose a weight that ensures you are not straining or compromising your form at any point during the exercise.

Don't be concerned about progressing in your weights. Choose a weight that you feel 110 percent comfortable lifting, or just use your body weight. Keep it light, and focus on simply moving that beautiful body of yours.

Take adequate rest in between each circuit to ensure that you could easily carry on a normal conversation while exercising. This may be as little as 30 seconds or up to a couple minutes of rest.

This program's exercises are to be completed as one large circuit. This means that you will complete all of

YOUR FIT THIRD TRIMESTER						
Day 1	Day 2	Day 3	Day 4	Day 5	Day 6	Day 7
Strength Train: full body	Cardio activity	Strength Train: upper body	Strength Train: lower body	Yoga / Stretch	Strength Train: full body	Cardio activity
Include at least three Core Confidence moves each day (chapter 3).						
If your schedule permits, add 20–30 minutes of walking or low-impact cardio activity.						

the exercises in the workout for the prescribed number of reps, rest, and then repeat all of the moves in the circuit. You continue this format until you've reached your target number of sets.

This large circuit style of workout will naturally force you to further decrease the amount of weight that you are lifting in each exercise compared to the workouts in the second trimester. This is for the safety of both you and baby.

Stop exercising if you feel you are pushing it. Some days are like that—always listen to your body.

BEGINNER: Complete 1–2 sets of each exercise for 12–15 repetitions. Choose a light weight or use your own body weight.

Finish your workout with a 15-minute walk.

INTERMEDIATE: Complete 2–3 sets of each exercise for 12–15 repetitions.

If performing 2 sets, then finish your workout with a 15-minute walk.

ADVANCED: Complete 3 sets of each exercise for 12–15 repetitions. Notice how the repetition range is the same as the intermediate exerciser. This is done on purpose as we want to keep the weight lighter in comparison to the first two trimesters.

CARDIO

The Basics:

Choose a low-impact activity that raises your heart rate slightly for 20–30 minutes, ensuring that you could easily carry on a normal conversation while exercising.

The activity does not need to be performed for a continuous 30 minutes. Two 15-minute sessions are equally as effective.

Remember that you are getting in cardiovascular benefits for you and baby during your strength training sessions, too!

Activity options for days 2 and 7:

- Walking
- Elliptical machine
- Stepper machine
- Swimming (use a flotation device such as a flutter board to help you swim)

DAY 1—STRENGTH TRAIN: FULL BODY

A1	A2	A3	B1	B2	B3
Front lunge	Cable front raise	Incline chest flye	Upright chest press	Cable pull-through*	Alternating dumbbell curl (seated)

*Alternate exercise is a seated hamstring curl. This machine is found at most gyms and is a great alternative for working the backs of your legs.

DAY 3—STRENGTH TRAINING: UPPER BODY

A1	A2	A3	A4	A5
Rope pull-down	Evil 18s	Cross-overs	Face pull with rope	Rear delt flye (standing wide legged)

DAY 4—STRENGTH TRAINING: LOWER BODY

A1	A2	A3	A4	A5
Glute bridge on BOSU	Leg extensions (toes out)	Lunge on BOSU	Side squat on BOSU	Wall sit (30-60 seconds)

DAY 6—STRENGTH TRAINING: FULL BODY

A1	A2	A3	A4	A5
Seated leg extension (toes straight)	Seated lateral raises	Curtsy lunge	Cable overhead rope extension	Rear delt cable pull

YOGA

This yoga-based sequence of five prenatal stretches and restorative poses takes you from standing to sitting to laying down.

Hold or gently move through each pose for 2–3 minutes, focusing on your breath.

Breathe slowly in and out through your nose.

Gently move your body through the full ranges of motion, never straining during a pose.

Repeat the sequence for a total of two sequences.

DAY 5—YOGA / STRETCH				
1	2	3	4	5
L-standing supported by wall	Cat/Cow	Child pose	Partner heart and butterfly	Reclining butterfly supported with pillows

" What Nobody Told Me "

STRENGTHENING AND REHABILITATING her pelvic floor is the most important thing a woman can do for her body before and after childbirth. Hands down. It's just as important as feeding and nurturing your newborn—it is something that must happen and is necessary for optimal pelvic health.

I learned this the hard way. Looking back on my experience, I wish someone had said this to me after the birth of my daughter. I was cleared to work out by my midwife at 6 weeks; however, she didn't do an internal exam, she didn't check on the status of my pelvic floor, no talk about the importance of letting it heal, or exercises I could do to strengthen it. Nothing. She checked my episiotomy scar and sent me on my way.

I was completely ignorant of the role the pelvic floor plays in pregnancy and childbirth. I had no idea the trauma it endures and the stress it takes on. I figured if I had been cleared to work out, everything must be fine. I knew things were stretched, and I knew my ligaments were looser then normal, but I had no idea that my pelvic organs could shift, that they could fall out of place, that they could prolapse. I had no idea because it was never discussed, it was never brought up, and it was never addressed. I was told to do Kegels, but I thought that was just so I wouldn't pee myself later in life. If I had been told that I would be diagnosed with a pelvic organ prolapse (POP) six weeks after the birth of my daughter, you can guarantee that I would have done whatever it took to avoid it.

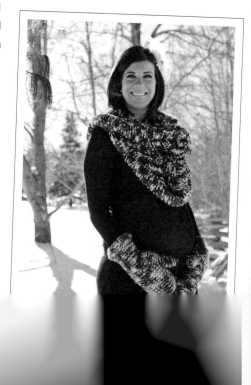

I went to the gym the day I was cleared by my midwife. I threw some weights around, did a little high-intensity interval training (HIIT), and I thought I was doing my body good. I was so proud of myself for getting back into it so soon. I was going to be an inspiration for women, someone new moms looked up to. I was going to get my body back in record time. It wasn't until later that night that I found the lump in my vagina that would change my life forever.

There is no cure for POP—once you have it, you live with it. It isn't life threatening, but it does greatly affect your quality of life and it certainly can influence your state of mind. The happiest months of my life as a new mom, cuddling my baby girl, were also my darkest. In my mind, my body had failed me as it created a miracle and then it let me down. I went from being someone who worked out six times a week to not even being able to walk without being uncomfortable. I could hold my baby standing still, but was advised not to pick her up, carry her, or bounce her for prolonged periods. I was told to avoid stairs, not to lift anything heavier than my baby (so I couldn't lift her in her car seat), and to do Kegels. I used to be an athlete and now I can't even walk. I felt broken, I felt lost, and I felt alone.

I was so used to being active that being told not to do things did not resonate well with me. So I did my research. I became an expert on pelvic organ prolapse. I was constantly researching; every chance I got I read about POP. I learned how to strengthen my body so I could be active again, and I learned what I needed to do to get my body back. I found a ton of resources that guided me and helped me understand how to work with my body. I had to accept my new normal and accept the fact that my body had changed. I know now what I can do and what I shouldn't do. The common theme in all my readings was to strengthen and rehab the pelvic floor, to ensure the core was strong and "on."

Because of what I've learned and experienced, I cannot stress enough the importance of rehabilitating your pelvic floor. That should be the *first* thing you do as a new mom, before you go back to the gym, before you start to lift, and most definitely before you start any high-impact exercise of any kind. You may feel fine, but trust me, your insides may not be—even if you're "super fit gal." It takes time for your body to completely heal after pregnancy and childbirth. It does some of the work itself, but you need to help it along the way. If you are active or want to be in the future, it is a no-brainer. You need to do the work and strengthen it. I'm eleven months postpartum now and I still work on strengthening my pelvic floor every single day, and I will continue to do so for the rest of my life.

POP won't happen to everyone, but rushing into exercise too fast, too soon could heighten your chances of getting it or other pelvic floor disorders. Diastis recti and incontinence are also linked to poor pelvic floor heath.

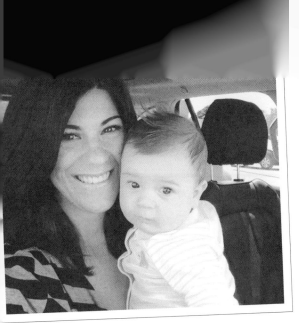

I am back to working out now, but that didn't come fast, and it certainly didn't come easy. Here is a snapshot of how I progressed with my workouts. My recovery was a lot longer because of my condition. Not everyone will take this long because not everyone will have a prolapse. However, regardless of your situation, it is important to take it slow. Don't start out too heavy or too high impact. Be kind to your body! It's not a race. You will regret it if you push yourself too hard too soon.

Rehabilitate your pelvic floor. Take the time to do this and make sure you see it through. Do your exercises for at least 4–6 weeks, three times a week.

Give yourself time and find a program that is progressive. Do not rush into anything and do not start with HIIT as your first workout. Start with low-impact exercise. Walking can be a great workout, and you can take baby with you. I started with 10-minute walks several times a day until I could walk a total of 30 minutes without feeling uncomfortable. This took me at least six months.

Once I could walk and felt a bit stronger down below, I started using bands to wake up my muscles. I did high reps to feel the burn.

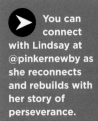

> You can connect with Lindsay at @pinkernewby as she reconnects and rebuilds with her story of perseverance.

After the bands, I used 5- to 8-pound weights until I was strong enough to complete 3 sets with 15 reps. While using the weights I did a Kegel with each repetition and held my inner core (transverse abdominals) tight. I continue to progress to heavier weights monthly, yet the important thing for me to remember is form: keeping my inner core tight and pulling up and in while performing a strong Kegel.

If at any time I feel like I am holding my breath or increasing my inner abdominal pressure too much, I stop what I am doing immediately. I still make sure to do my pelvic exercises 3–4 times a week, and often I'll do them in between sets if time allows.

Pregnancy is no joke: It wreaks havoc on your body. Things shift, things stretch, and things are weakened. Take it from someone who has lived it: Do not rush into anything; take your time getting back into exercise. Be kind to your body and don't set any unrealistic expectations. Enjoy your time with your baby—enjoy being a mom.

MY FIT BUMP

THIRD TRIMESTER (28 WEEKS)

Place your photo here

MY FIT BUMP

THIRD TRIMESTER (32 WEEKS)

Place your photo here

MY FIT BUMP

THIRD TRIMESTER (38 WEEKS)

Place your photo here

MY FIT THIRD TRIMESTER | NUTRITION

MY TYPICAL DAILY MENU

Breakfast _____

_____

❑ Water

Mid-morning _____

_____

❑ Water

Lunch _____

_____

❑ Water

Mid-afternoon _____

_____

❑ Water

Dinner _____

_____

❑ Water

Evening (optional) _____

_____

❑ Water

MY FIT THIRD TRIMESTER | NUTRITION

SHOPPING LIST

Lean Proteins

- ❑ _____
- ❑ _____
- ❑ _____
- ❑ _____

Complex Carbs

- ❑ _____
- ❑ _____
- ❑ _____
- ❑ _____

Fruits & Veggies

- ❑ _____
- ❑ _____
- ❑ _____
- ❑ _____

Healthy Fats

- ❑ _____
- ❑ _____
- ❑ _____
- ❑ _____

MY FIT THIRD TRIMESTER

EXERCISE & TRACKING SHEET

EXERCISE NAME	MONTH 7 (REPS & LBS)	MONTH 8 (REPS & LBS)	MONTH 9 (REPS & LBS)

CORE CONFIDENCE TRACKER:

Put a checkmark below each time you strengthen your core & pelvic floor.

❑ ❑ ❑ ❑ ❑ ❑ ❑ ❑ ❑ ❑ ❑

CARDIO

Note your cardio activity this trimester:

_____

_____

_____

MY FIT THIRD TRIMESTER

EXERCISE & TRACKING SHEET

EXERCISE NAME	MONTH 7 (REPS & LBS)	MONTH 8 (REPS & LBS)	MONTH 9 (REPS & LBS)

CORE CONFIDENCE TRACKER:

Put a checkmark below each time you strengthen your core & pelvic floor.

❏ ❏ ❏ ❏ ❏ ❏ ❏ ❏ ❏ ❏ ❏ ❏

CARDIO

Note your cardio activity this trimester:

_____

_____

_____

MY FIT THIRD TRIMESTER

EXERCISE & TRACKING SHEET

EXERCISE NAME	MONTH 7 (REPS & LBS)	MONTH 8 (REPS & LBS)	MONTH 9 (REPS & LBS)

CORE CONFIDENCE TRACKER:

Put a checkmark below each time you strengthen your core & pelvic floor.

❑ ❑ ❑ ❑ ❑ ❑ ❑ ❑ ❑ ❑ ❑

CARDIO

Note your cardio activity this trimester:

_____

_____

_____

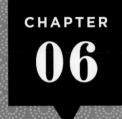

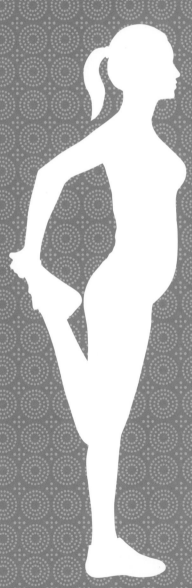

YOUR FIT POST-BABY: BUILDING TO LAST

→ Hello mommy! Have you thought of post-partum as your "fourth trimester"? It's a time period like no other, so let's take your amazing body forward by building it to last!

You made it! Baby has arrived!!! Congratulations, you (finally!) get to snuggle your little baby bundle. I had a beautiful baby girl and we named her Faith. Baby Faith was flopped on top of my chest, covered in the mess of afterbirth, weighing a healthy 8 pounds, 5 ounces. I was in love.

Though as much as we love our babies, it certainly isn't all baby bliss, right? You're probably wondering, *What now?* Even though you did your best to stay fit during your pregnancy, you may glance down at your bulging tummy and thick thighs and think about getting back into shape fast!

Hold up! "Wait six weeks and you're okay" is not accurate general advice. Your body has just gone through major trauma. Yes, I know that *trauma* is a strong word, but the impact on your body of growing and birthing a baby is significant. Did you know that your internal organs can fall out postpartum? Whether you delivered vaginally or by C-section, it took 9 months for your body to adapt and change. Do you think that it's realistic that 6 weeks is all it takes to heal? And while you stayed fit during your fit pregnancy, your body is still human. Trying to prove you are superhuman is not something to be admired, but has the potential

to leave you with a long-term negative impact.

I understand the allure of wanting to race to get back in shape. That baby bump you're still sporting post-baby doesn't look quite so adorable now, does it? Your clothes don't fit and you may be feeling *f-a-t*. Postpartum I was more than 20 pounds heavier than my pre-baby weight. I certainly wasn't fitting into my skinny jeans! My 4-year-old son regularly asked if I still had a baby in my belly. He commented on my big belly (a lot!).

As I coach my clients through their progressions, I tell them that a key aspect of moving forward is accepting where you are *now*. This is no different. With baby in tow, I went to the discount retail store and bought a few tops that fit and flattered me now. The lights in the changing room were not flattering, and the fit failed more than it worked, but rushing and dreaming of the future you steals joy from you today.

Your Fit Post-Baby Exercise

It's common to hear moms talking about "getting back" to a weight or shape they had pre-baby. Instead of "going back," I want to shift your mind to viewing your post-baby exercise plan as a plan centered on rehabilitation. While "rehabilitation" isn't the sexiest word for regaining your shape, it's a smarter approach, as it comes to having a body that lasts.

Your Post-Baby Plan: Built to Last

Do you want to be a strong mommy for life? Then you need a "built to last" plan, not a "get back into shape as fast as possible" plan. So where do you start to build to last?

1. Start slow and easy. **Don't jump, run, or pound yourself. Go for gentle walks pushing the baby stroller. You carried baby for nine months, and that put an incredible amount of strain on your pelvic floor. Even if you had a C-section, your pelvic floor needs rehabilitation.**

2. No high-intensity sessions **in your living room or boot camps. Even if you're "super fit gal," you need rehabilitation. Elite athletes get injured and do rehabilitation—why do you think you can skip this? Instead revisit chapter 3 and start with the Core Breath. The Core Breath is one of the first exercises you can do in the days following baby's birth to start the process of restoring your inner core. As long as you don't have complications,**

you can progress each week by adding one Core Confidence exercise to your routine. If you had any complications during pregnancy or after, send the Bellies Inc. team a message and confirm that the exercises are appropriate for you. Remember, all eight Core Confidence exercises from the Bellies Inc. team are at www. sisinshape.com under Shop.

3. Do not crunch. **As our tummies are healing (and even long after), your abs may be separated. Remember diastasis recti? This is the term for separation of your rectus abdominis. Performing a crunch motion with exposed organs pushes everything inside out. You are actually making your tummy worse! The Core Confidence exercises get your pelvic floor and your abdominals working together without crunching.**

4. At 6–8 weeks postpartum, **make an appointment with a pelvic floor physiotherapist to get a thorough assessment of the pelvic floor and checked for diastasis recti. This is important so she can prevent your going ahead with exercise that may result in incontinence, or pelvic organ prolapse, or may make ab separation worse.**

5. Stay progressive with your programs. The pelvic floor takes 3–6 months (or longer!) to heal, so you need to take small steps getting back into fitness. Again, no boot camps or high-intensity pounding, jumping, or jacking. Treat yourself like a beginner exerciser even if you worked out during your pregnancy. Don't focus on what you can't do; focus on what you can do! I love strength training, but even months after baby I treated myself like a beginner. I started at one set of basic stationary moves with light weights. I did not push through my pelvic floor or strain in any lifts. I kept my transverse abs engaged at all times, and when at any point I felt my inner core give out, I stopped the exercise immediately. Without an engaged and protected core, it was game over. I'd lighten the load or give it a rest and stick to walking. I was building to last and building to be a strong mom for life.

What Is Prolapse?

Pelvic organ prolapse is a type of pelvic floor dysfunction. Pelvic organs such as your bladder, uterus, small bowel, and rectum can prolapse by descending into or outside the vaginal canal or rectum. Early stage prolapse can show no symptoms or may present the following symptoms:

PELVIC PAIN

- A feeling of heaviness in lower abs
- Back pain
- Pulling sensation
- Discomfort during sex
- Incontinence

As the descent of the organs continues, symptoms may progress to the point where you feel like something is falling out, such as a tampon, or a bulging sensation in your vagina or heaviness that gets worse throughout the day.

Early detection is key, and it is critical that you see a pelvic floor physiotherapist, ideally during your pregnancy and at 6 weeks postpartum, for a full assessment. Your therapist will examine the pelvic floor and the internal organs to see if they are where they should be and if the muscles have the strength and endurance to support them. With that knowledge you will then know the best restorative exercises to do, what activities to avoid, and what steps to take to help prevent any conditions from getting any worse.

Revisiting Ab Separation: Diastasis Recti

We talked about diastasis recti in chapter 3, calling it "mummy tummy." We incorporated certain exercises in *Your Fit Pregnancy* to strengthen your inner core to help prevent ab separation. However, postpartum, we need to continue to work on rehabilitating our core, because diastasis is most commonly seen after pregnancy when your abdominal wall is lax.

Diastatis is thought to happen in 30–67 percent of pregnant women. That means diastasis happens a lot! Diastatis is more than just an aesthetic issue, because it reduces the integrity and function of your abdominal wall. This can result in low back pain, disc hernias, inability to lift heavy objects, and pelvic instability. If it's not addressed after your first pregnancy, then it may make pushing more difficult in your next pregnancy. So, as you're contemplating getting back to fit, your core integrity should be paramount, whatever activity you choose, whether it's running, strength training, playing tennis, or swinging around your kids.

To check if you have diastasis recti and how severe it is, there is a simple test you can perform on yourself, or you can see an experienced professional to do the test. As Julia from Bellies Inc. explains, "The test itself is stressful to the tissues and can cause damage. The real information comes at 8 weeks postpartum, as research shows that no further

improvement will occur with diastasis without intervention." So in the first 8 weeks treat yourself as if you have diastasis and pelvic floor dysfunction and take things slowly and avoid straining.

I want to make sure you are doing the self-assessment test properly, and I can do that more effectively in a video. I have a video by Samantha from Bellies Inc. explaining step-by-step how to correctly perform the diastasis self-assessment on my YouTube channel under the playlist "Post Partum Ab Rehab" (link to my YouTube feed at www.sisinshape.com).

How much of an ab separation is normal? As Julia from Bellies Inc. explains, "There is no data for optimal distance. Getting tension is most important, but generally two fingers of separation is 'normal,' as that's approximately one inch. However, it's not enough to just focus on the distance 'gap,' but also notice if you're creating tension across that space." Julia explains further, "I have seen three and four finger separations generate beautiful tension, and I have seen one finger separations have no tension at all." A lack of ability to create tension and/or a gap of more than 2.5 finger widths in the test is a sign of diastasis. If at any time you see a round, hard, or painful bulge protruding from your belly button area, or along your linea alba, then consult your doctor immediately.

Can the gap be closed and tension restored? The good news is yes, and it's never too late! No surgery is required; instead you need consistent proper ab rehab work (see the chapter 3 Core Confidence exercises), proper posture, and being mindful of your core throughout your daily movements. Whew! That's a lot of work. Yes, I get that it's not easy. I admit that I would have preferred to be doing bicep curls or sleeping, but I knew the ab gap would not fix itself, so I prioritized the exercises at the start of my workouts and did a couple more in the evening before bed. It was important that I engaged my linea alba throughout my entire day, not just during exercise. Picking up baby Faith and reaching to the bottom shelf were opportunities to protect and strengthen my inner core. And proper posture? I'd often catch myself with incorrect posture where I'd be standing or sitting slouched with my tailbone tucked in. I'd take a breath and then correct my posture so my pelvis was stacked and the bottom of my ribs lined up with the top of my hipbones.

Does this seem overwhelming? I felt it was at the beginning—we all have so much on our mind. But

taking one movement at a time and being more mindful made the biggest difference. As the weeks passed, this way of moving, exercising, and holding my posture became second nature. We're building to last, remember?

Your Fit Post-Baby Nutrition

After baby is born, feeding yourself may not seem as important, but what you eat plays a big role in your energy and recovery. Also, if you're breastfeeding, your body is providing the nourishment for your new arrival.

Food in the First Days after Baby

Post-baby, we experience a lot of nether-region issues, so ensuring our digestive health is top-notch will make the world of difference. That first poop is something I still try to block from my memory!

Of course we are grateful for our precious babies, but (ouch) vaginal tearing and hemorrhoids do not mix well with a bunged-up pooper. Fiber is the key remedy here, and while it's tempting to sprinkle on the All-Bran Buds or mix the Metamucil, the best bet for your tummy is fiber-rich foods, mostly in the form of fruits and vegetables. In the first days after baby, be sure to incorporate fiber-rich foods in your diet such as:

- Kale (any leafy greens do the trick)
- Broccoli
- Apples and pears
- Ground flaxseed (great in oatmeal and smoothies)
- Whole grain rice and bread
- Oatmeal
- Quinoa
- Fruits

There are also a number of other solutions to help your digestive health:

- Drinking lots of water. Hydration helps!
- Being active. Get your digestive pipes pumping by getting up for a walk or two each day.
- Drinking hot lemon water.

But What about Losing This Weight?

Ah, yes. Shedding the baby weight. Couldn't *all* that extra weight just come out with the baby? We've established that now is not the time to join a bootcamp for your physical well-being. It's also not the time to jump into a diet. When it comes to weight loss, let's first be realistic and manage our expectations. We have a newborn to care for, our sleep is a mess, and adding the expectation of rapid weight loss to our plate is simply too much pressure. Slim and

trim with a newborn on our hip— it's that unattainable ideal state that gets too many of us women feeling like we're not enough or less than adequate. So first let's ditch the time line!

There is a lot you can do to move toward a healthier you, which always has a by-product of you looking your best! The nutrition (not *diet*) in this book for pregnancy is ideal for postpartum, too. The three fundamentals are the same:

1. Ensure you are getting a balance of all the macronutrients (carbohydrates, proteins, and fats).

2. Drink plenty of plain, pure water.

3. Fill your plate and nosh on micronutrients (foods rich in vitamins and minerals).

After baby Faith was born, I was finally relieved of all of my food aversions and found that by simply incorporating better food choices, in appropriate portions from the Handy Portion Sizes guidelines, some of the excess weight came off easily.

Breastfeeding may or may not help you lose weight. Many women find that until they are done breastfeeding, the last 5–10 pounds will not come off due to hormones, while other women find they can't keep enough weight on while breastfeeding.

The nutrition in this book is an incredible first step in creating lasting healthy habits. My postpartum clients first follow the fundamentals in this book, walk daily, perform their Core Confidence exercises, and start some very basic beginner-level strength training. All have success at shedding some of the excess weight and are setting themselves up to build a lasting and strong body. However, if you've mastered all this and you are at a point where you really want to shed some more of the excess baby weight, then consider these tips:

Sustainable fat loss seems to elude the majority of people trying to lose weight. Seek out sustainable and gradual methods to increase your chances of keeping the weight off. If you can't see yourself following the nutrition program for maintaining your weight, then it's likely not a good choice for long-term fat loss.

Are there extra treats in your diet? A maintenance plan for my clients includes a couple treat meals a week where you don't pay attention to quality macronutrient choices— you just enjoy the meal! However, when it comes to weight loss, consider reducing the treat meals to one or eliminating them for a couple weeks.

Portion size check. Ensure your portions are following the visuals shown in the Handy Portion Sizes guide. To lose weight gradually, simply reduce these portion sizes a bit. This doesn't require you to vastly change your diet or eliminate any foods.

Weight loss is never easy. You can start out with a truckload of good intentions, then life happens. Birthday parties, sick family members, baby's sleeping sucks, returning to work, and *life*! Life will happen, which means you will stumble, but accept each failure as a learning opportunity. What healthier solutions can you use the next time life happens? We'll be successful if we *fail forward*. Get help if you need it; if you want to change, then change. But be patient and be kind to yourself in the process.

Breastfeeding

I breastfed baby Faith, so I needed to ensure I was getting sufficient energy from food to produce milk. This is important especially in the first 6 weeks as your milk supply is being established. You need 400–500 additional calories to support breastfeeding. I followed a meal plan similar to that in trimester 3 to ensure I was getting sufficient energy to make baby's milk. I also ate a few additional small snacks whenever I was hungry (sometimes in the middle of the night!). The focus was on choosing quality macronutrients, in appropriate portions, that were loaded with power micronutrients. Also, water intake is critical for your milk supply, so be sure you're sipping water all day long—at minimum, 3 liters!

As women continue to recover from their pregnancies and are incorporating more exercise into their routines, most ask me about whether their milk supply will be impacted. As long as you are eating sufficient calories and your milk supply is established, exercise will not impact your milk supply. That said, extreme exercise or drastically slashing calories could impact your milk supply, and that's one more reason I don't recommend either of those.

Can you safely take a protein powder while you are breastfeeding? The same guidance applies as when you are pregnant, so hop back to the section in chapter 2 to review those guidelines.

Let's Go Forward, Not "Back"!

It's popular for people to say after baby that they're "back" to their pre-pregnancy shape and weight (or trying to get "back"). One afternoon while nursing Faith, I saw her tiny feet nestled under my flabby tummy and it struck me: *I don't ever want to go back. I'm only going forward.* Trying to go "back" seemed disrespectful to the blessing of her in my life.

It all came flooding in with that thought—there is no room for (self-) hate in a full heart. Since that day, I've changed my language to "going forward." That shift in language and mentality has made this postpartum journey one of love instead of one propelled by dislike. Our bodies have been stretched to the max, but so have our hearts and sense of self. You don't go back, you go forward from that. So let's go forward—here's to being strong mommies and women for life!

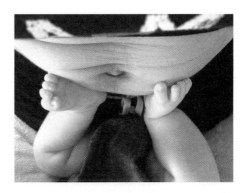

"I Love the Woman I've Become"

"I LOVE THE WOMAN I'VE BECOME, because I've fought to become her." To me, that quote sums up the images of me you see here. You see me holding my sweet baby, but I wonder if you can see what this image represents, as there is so much more going on in that photo than meets the eye.

What you can't see is the self-acceptance that took place to acquire the courage for these photos. Owning my 4-month post-baby body. Why does it feel like a race to the finish line to lose those pregnancy pounds or button those pre-pregnancy pants? It's a race against whom, for whom, and what's the finish line?

We all see the tabloids. "Look how fast Kim Kardashian lost *all that baby weight*!" or "She got her bikini body back in 12 weeks!"

Having had three babies, I understand the dream so many women have, that once the baby is just 12 weeks old, we step back out into the world fresh faced, well rested, and ready for a bikini—as if the stork brought the baby to the doorstep.

Well, that hasn't been the case for me, and I know it's not the case for most women. So why do we let our minds think this way? Are we scared that if we haven't gotten there in 12 weeks we won't ever get there?

It seems to me that we women often put unrealistic pressure on ourselves to look a certain way during pregnancy and after having a baby. We compare ourselves to a magazine cover or a close friend who left the hospital in her skinny jeans. Wouldn't it be nice if we gave ourselves a little leeway and longer time frames for getting the body back and were just concerned about providing a healthy pregnancy and life for our new blessing?

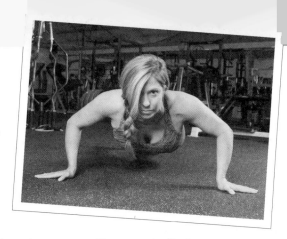

So here I am, 4 months post-partum, at a photo shoot. I knew about this photo shoot shortly after baby was born, and while I wanted to look amazing (what woman wouldn't?), I also wanted to look real, and *Gorgo Women's Fitness Magazine* gave me the opportunity to be real. The magazine editor explained that *Gorgo* wanted to show fit women at all stages of life, and as a breastfeeding mom, I was certainly in a stage!

Nourishing my body to feed my baby was more of a priority than the few last pounds. I had lost some pregnancy weight because as soon as I could exercise, I put my energy and focus into making my body strong again. But considering that a year or so before these pictures I was a competitive physique athlete, this body is not the body I would have chosen for a photo shoot. I had to come to a place of self-acceptance.

I'm comfortable to say that I'm not worried about being skinny. I want a strong and healthy body, however long my fitness journey takes—a lifetime, I hope.

You can connect with Christie at fitnixfitness.com as this power mama honestly shares her journey to step into (and embrace) her strength.

So for this photo shoot, I am happy to say that I walked right up to that unrealistic finish line and stepped right over it. It will never be about the finish for me but the journey toward the strong body I am working to build. I continue to fight to be the woman I am becoming, the woman I know I will be, three kids and all, no matter how long it takes, the right way, the realistic way, to show women, moms, that we all have a journey and that postpartum progress takes time—and that's okay.

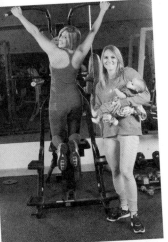

There was a time that I wouldn't have been able to stand in front of a camera not feeling my best or most beautiful. But being vulnerable enough to do so, owning where I am while I strive for more, is the woman I will forever fight to be.

MY FIT POST-BABY

MOMMY & BABY ❤

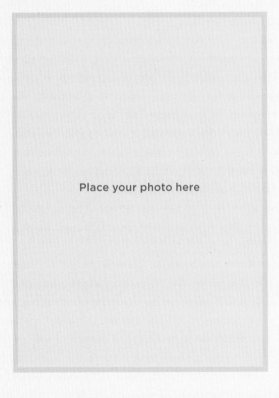

Place your photo here

MY (AMAZING) POST-BABY BODY

My favorite way to hold you in my strong arms is . . . _____
_____
_____

I carry you for _____ hours each day with my strong back supporting us.

Your strong heart sounds like _____ .

My favorite place my strong legs take us is _____ .

I watch you breathing and think _____
_____
_____ .

"Being a mother is about strengths you didn't know you had."

—LINDA WOOTEN

MY FIT POST-BABY

BUILT-TO-LAST CHECKLIST

❑ Start slow & easy. My favorite place to walk you in your stroller is _____
_____

❑ Core confidence rehabilitation program (chapter 3)

❑ Appointment with pelvic floor physiotherapist (6–8 weeks post-baby).
    ❑ Checked for diastasis recti
        ❑ Ab separation _____ inches
        ❑ Tension? Yes or No
    ❑ Checked strength of pelvic floor
        ❑ Exercises recommended by physiotherapist

❑ Appointment with doctor (6–8 weeks post-baby)

❑ I have a progressive fitness program appropriate for ME!

Notes: _____

_____

_____

_____

_____

_____

_____

_____

_____

_____

_____

_____

_____

_____

_____

_____

_____

_____

_____

_____

_____

_____

_____

_____

_____

_____

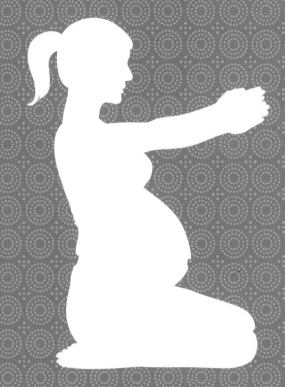

PREGGO POWER RECIPES

→ Food that nourishes, tastes yummy, and satisfies your cravings. It is possible for your pregnancy!

RECIPES BY: Christal Sczebel, Registered Holistic Nutritionist
www.nutritionistinthekitch.com

FOOD PHOTOGRAPHY: Christal Sczebel

CARROT CAKE OVERNIGHT OATS

Serves: 1

INGREDIENTS

- 1/3 cup rolled oats
- 1 tablespoon ground flaxseed
- 1/4 teaspoon ground cinnamon
- 1/8 teaspoon ground nutmeg
- 1–2 packets stevia (or 5 drops liquid stevia)
- 1/4 cup raw shredded carrot
- 2 tablespoons chopped pineapple
- 1 tablespoon shredded unsweetened coconut
- 1/4 teaspoon pure vanilla extract
- 1/2 cup unsweetened almond milk (plus more if needed for serving)

INSTRUCTIONS

1. In a bowl combine all ingredients and mix well.

2. Cover and place in the refrigerator overnight.

3. In the morning, stir the mixture and add 1–2 tablespoons of almond milk or water. Heat in the microwave or on the stovetop or enjoy cold!

NUTRITIONAL INFORMATION: Calories: 224 kcal; Fat: 7 g; Carbohydrates: 30 g; Protein: 0 g

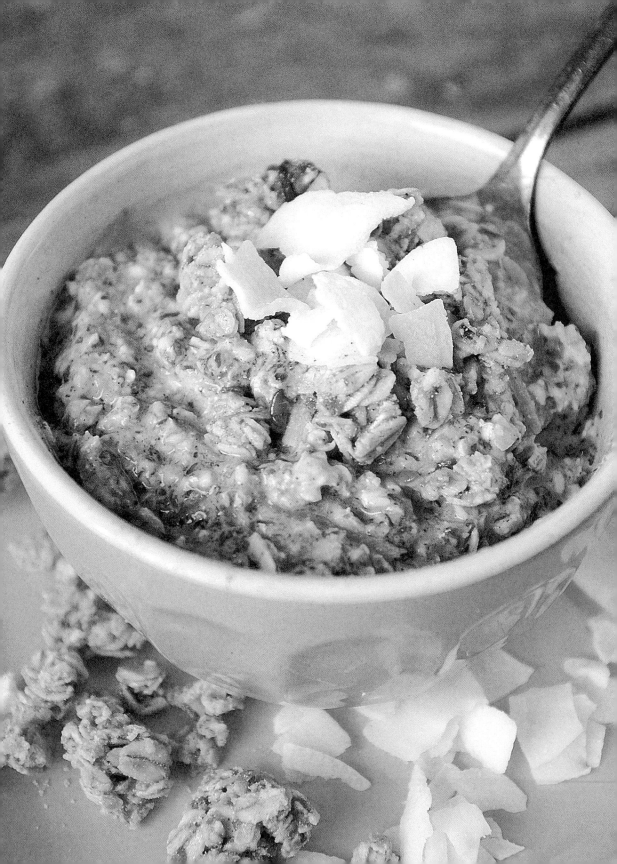

FRUIT-FILLED
OVERNIGHT QUINOA AND OATS

Serves: 1

INGREDIENTS

¼ cup large flaked rolled oats

¼ cup cooked quinoa

½ tablespoon ground flaxseed

1 teaspoon cinnamon

1 packet stevia (or 5 drops liquid stevia)

¼ banana, mashed

2 tablespoons raspberries

2 tablespoons blueberries

¼ cup diced peaches

8 almonds

¾ cup unsweetened almond milk

INSTRUCTIONS

1. In a medium bowl combine the oats, quinoa, ground flaxseed, cinnamon, and stevia. Stir to combine.

2. Add the mashed banana, raspberries, blueberries, peaches, and almonds.

3. Pour in the almond milk, and mix ingredients together.

4. Place in the fridge and leave overnight.

5. In the morning, remove from the fridge and heat on the stovetop or microwave, or enjoy cold! If you find the mixture is too thick in the morning, just add some water.

NUTRITIONAL INFORMATION: Calories: 295 kcal; Fat: 11 g; Carbohydrates: 44 g; Protein: 11 g

COCONUT FLOUR APPLE PANCAKES

Serves: 1

INGREDIENTS

3 tablespoons coconut flour

1 tablespoon ground flaxseed

1/2 teaspoon baking powder

1/8 teaspoon salt

1/2 teaspoon cinnamon

1 packet stevia (or 5 drops)

3/4 cup egg whites

1 tablespoon plain almond milk

1 tablespoon unsweetened applesauce

1/4 teaspoon pure vanilla extract

1/4 apple thinly sliced

1/2 tablespoon pure maple syrup

INSTRUCTIONS

1. In a large bowl combine the coconut flour, flaxseed, baking powder, salt, cinnamon, and stevia (if using a liquid sweetener, wait and combine with the wet ingredients).

2. In a separate bowl combine the eggs, almond milk, applesauce, and vanilla.

3. Adding small amounts at a time, combine the wet ingredients with the dry until all is incorporated.

4. Allow the batter to sit for 1 to 2 minutes.

5. Heat a nonstick skillet to medium heat (spray lightly with olive oil spray if needed).

6. Once heated, add in batter (about 2 tablespoons for each pancake).

7. Wait a minute or so and top the pancake with an apple slice (the pancake should be partly cooked at this point and the apple slice will sit nicely on top).

8. Flip each pancake only when the edges are fully cooked; cook for an additional 2 minutes on the opposite side.

9. Repeat until you are out of batter.

10. Top the pancakes with pure maple syrup.

NUTRITIONAL INFORMATION: Calories: 263 kcal; Fat: 5g; Carbohydrates: 30g; Protein: 25g

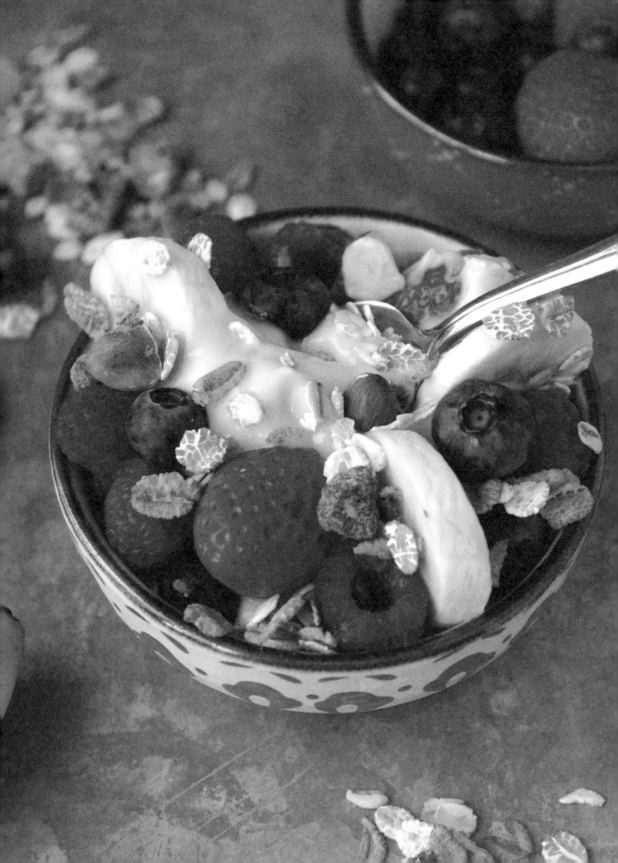

BREAKFAST MUESLI BOWL

Serves: 1

INGREDIENTS

- 1 cup plain 0% fat Greek yogurt
- 1/2 banana, sliced
- 1/2 cup frozen or fresh berries
- 1/4 cup unsweetened muesli
- 1/2 tablespoon chia seeds
- 1 teaspoon honey or pure maple syrup

INSTRUCTIONS

1. Place the yogurt in a bowl.

2. Top with the sliced banana and berries.

3. Sprinkle with the muesli and chia seeds.

4. Drizzle lightly with honey or pure maple syrup.

5. Devour!

NUTRITIONAL INFORMATION: Calories: 300 kcal; Fat: 3 g; Carbohydrates: 40 g; Protein: 25 g

EASY ITALIAN BAKED EGGS

Serves: 1

INGREDIENTS

1/2 teaspoon olive oil

2 tablespoons diced onion

1 1/2 cups fresh spinach

1/4 cup prepared marinara sauce

1 large organic egg

1/3 cup egg whites

1/4 cup mozzarella, shredded

2 tablespoons light Parmesan cheese

1/4 teaspoon Italian seasoning

dash of salt

dash of pepper

INSTRUCTIONS

1. Preheat the oven to 400 degrees F.

2. Add the oil to a saucepan and heat on medium. Add the onions and sauté until soft, about 3 minutes.

3. Add the spinach and sauté until just wilted, about 2 minutes.

4. Stir in the marinara sauce and sauté until heated through.

5. Transfer the mixture to a ceramic soup bowl or individual-sized ramekin.

6. Crack in the egg and pour in the egg whites.

7. Top with mozzarella and Parmesan cheese and sprinkle with Italian seasoning, salt, and pepper.

8. Bake for 10 minutes, then broil for an additional 2 minutes until the cheese is bubbling.

NUTRITIONAL INFORMATION: Calories: 230 kcal; Fat: 10 g; Carbohydrates: 8 g; Fiber: 3 g; Protein: 24 g

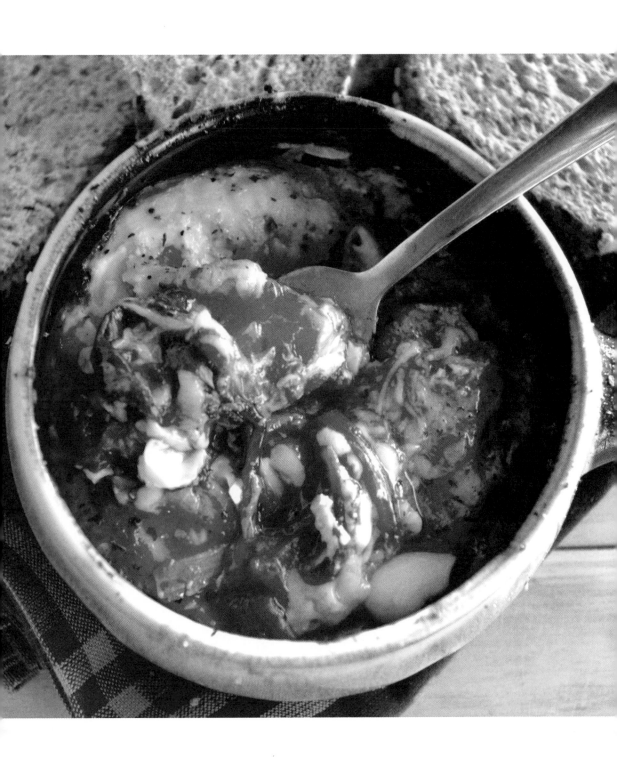

PUMPKIN GRANOLA YOGURT PARFAIT

Serves: 1

INGREDIENTS

- ¼ cup canned pure pumpkin purée
- 1 tablespoon pure maple syrup
- ¼ teaspoon ground nutmeg
- ½ teaspoon ground cinnamon
- 1 cup plain 0% Greek yogurt
- 2 tablespoons pumpkin granola (Nature's Path brand suggested)

INSTRUCTIONS

1. Add the pumpkin, maple syrup, nutmeg, and cinnamon to a bowl and mix until well combined.

2. Pour half the pumpkin mixture into a parfait glass or bowl, then layer with half the yogurt, the rest of the pumpkin mixture, then the rest of the yogurt. Chill for 10–30 minutes.

3. Once chilled, top with the granola.

Make It Quick Tip: Mix all ingredients together and enjoy!

NUTRITIONAL INFORMATION: Calories: 254 kcal; Fat: 3 g; Carbohydrates: 33 g; Protein: 26 g

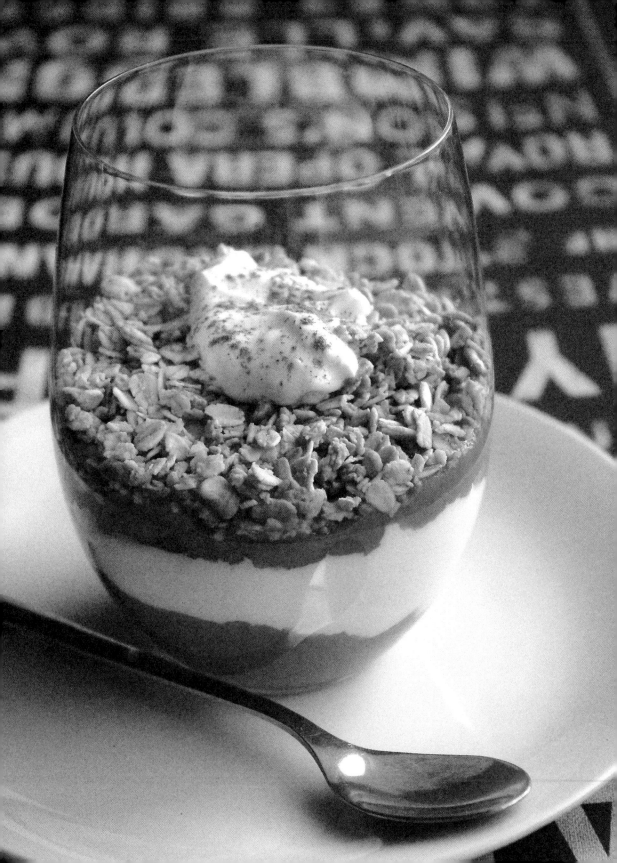

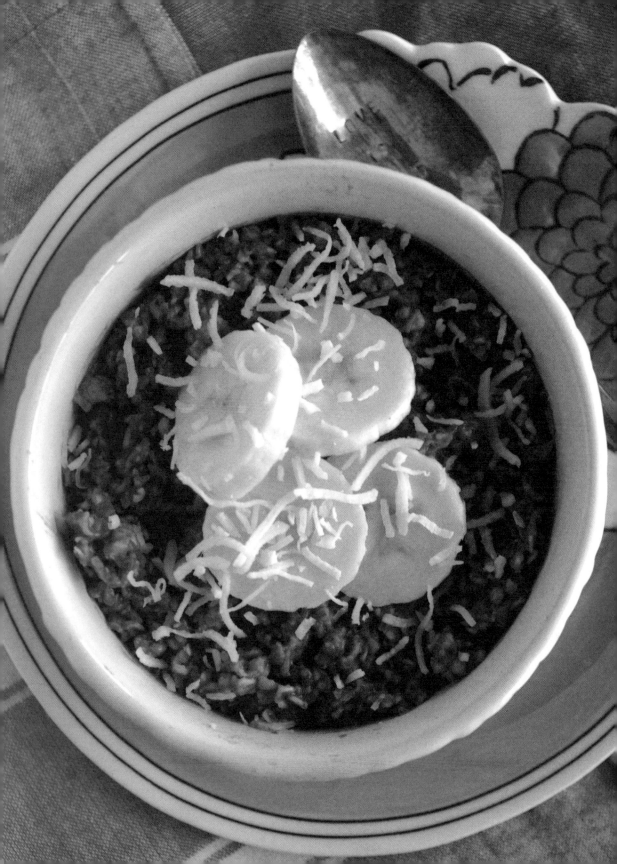

CHUNKY MONKEY OATMEAL

Serves: 1

INGREDIENTS

- ½ cup instant oats (gluten-free if needed)
- chocolate-flavored stevia to taste (or 5 drops liquid stevia and 1 teaspoon cocoa powder)
- ½ cup unsweetened chocolate almond milk (or plain unsweetened almond milk with just enough chocolate-flavored stevia or cocoa powder added to get a nice chocolate taste)
- ½ cup water
- a few slices of banana (about ⅛ of a banana)
- 1 tablespoon shredded unsweetened coconut

INSTRUCTIONS

1. Place the oats and stevia in a bowl and stir to combine.

2. In a small pot, bring the almond milk and water to a boil.

3. Once boiling, add the almond milk and water mixture to the oat mixture and cover for 5 minutes.

4. Slice the banana and stir it into the oatmeal.

5. Top with shredded coconut.

6. Enjoy!

NUTRITIONAL INFORMATION: Calories: 180 kcal; Fat: 7 g; Carbohydrates: 34 g; Protein: 0 g

PB&J PROTEIN BARS

Serves: 6

INGREDIENTS

- 3/4 cup pitted dates
- 1/4 cup whole raw peanuts
- 3 scoops no-additives, naturally sweetened whey isolate or whey concentrate
- 1/2 cup unsweetened dried cranberries
- 1/4 cup natural peanut butter
- 3 tablespoons unsweetened almond milk (plus more if needed)

INSTRUCTIONS

1. Soak the dates in warm water for 15 minutes, then drain.

2. Place the peanuts and whey in a food processor and process for 30 seconds.

3. Add in the dates, cranberries, peanut butter, and almond milk. Process again until well combined and a sticky batter is achieved.

4. Scoop the mixture into a square baking pan and firmly press down to make an even layer.

5. Place in the freezer for 30 minutes to set, then cut into 6 bars.

6. Store in the freezer or fridge.

NUTRITIONAL INFORMATION: Per 1 Bar: Calories: 245 kcal; Fat: 7 g; Carbohydrates: 29 g; Protein: 20 g

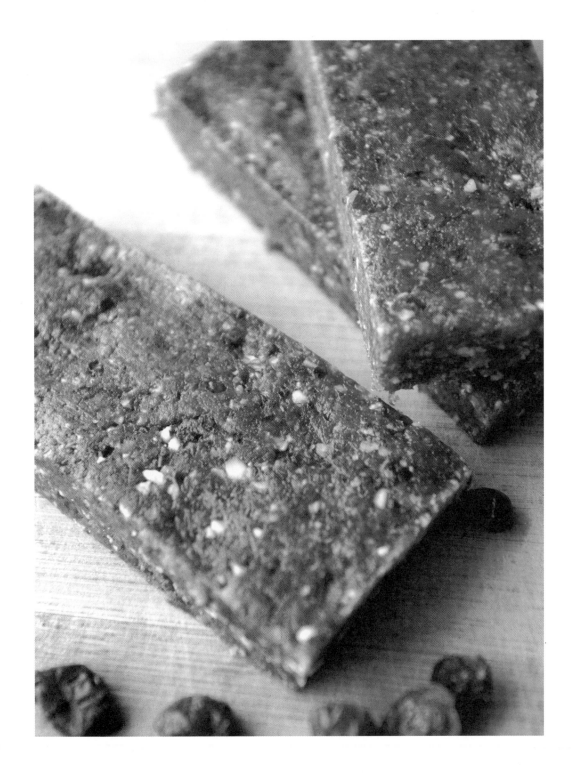

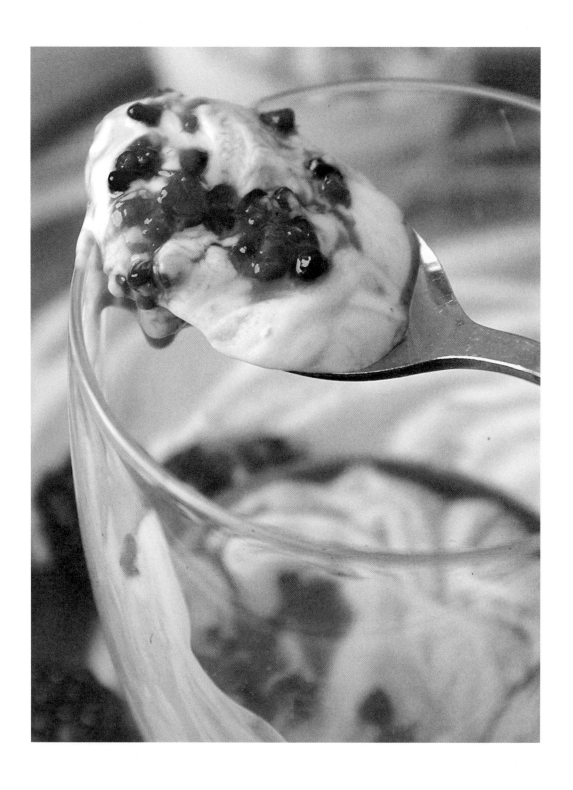

BLACKBERRY MAPLE
ALMOND BUTTER GREEK YOGURT

Serves: 1

INGREDIENTS

- 1 cup plain 0% Greek yogurt
- 1 packet stevia (or 5 drops liquid stevia)
- ½ tablespoon natural almond butter
- ½ cup fresh blackberries
- 2 teaspoons pure maple syrup

INSTRUCTIONS

1. Mix the yogurt, stevia, and almond butter in a bowl.

2. Add the blackberries and drizzle with maple syrup.

NUTRITIONAL INFORMATION: Calories: 240 kcal; Fat: 6 g; Carbohydrates: 23 g; Protein: 26 g

PEACH COBBLER GREEK YOGURT

Serves: 1

INGREDIENTS

- 1 cup plain 0% Greek yogurt (250 grams)
- 1 packet stevia (or 5 drops liquid stevia)
- 1 teaspoon cinnamon
- 1 teaspoon natural almond butter
- ⅓ cup finely diced peaches
- 2 tablespoons rolled oats or muesli

INSTRUCTIONS

1. Mix the yogurt, stevia, cinnamon, and almond butter in a bowl.

2. Add the diced peaches and sprinkle with the oats.

NUTRITIONAL INFORMATION: Calories: 240 kcal; Fat: 4 g; Carbohydrates: 23 g; Protein: 26 g

STRAWBERRY KIWI CHIA GREEK YOGURT

Serves: 1

INGREDIENTS

- 1 cup plain 0% Greek yogurt (250 grams)
- 1 packet stevia (or 5 drops liquid stevia)
- 1 tablespoon black chia seeds
- 4 diced strawberries
- ½ small kiwi, diced

INSTRUCTIONS

1. Mix the yogurt, stevia, and chia seeds.

2. Top with strawberries and kiwi.

NUTRITIONAL INFORMATION: Calories: 250 kcal; Fat: 7 g; Carbohydrates: 22 g; Protein: 28 g

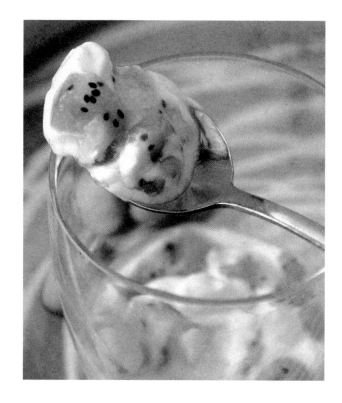

EASY EGG MUFFINS

Serves: 4 (3 muffins each serving)

INGREDIENTS

olive oil spray

4 scallions (or green onions), minced

2 large carrots, shredded

1 red bell pepper, minced

3 cups egg whites

4 whole eggs

1 teaspoon basil

dash of sea salt and pepper

1/4 cup shredded mozzarella cheese

INSTRUCTIONS

1. Preheat oven to 375 degrees F.

2. Coat a large 12-muffin or two large 6-muffin tins with a small amount of olive oil spray to prevent sticking.

3. Combine the scallions, carrots, and bell pepper in a bowl. Fill each muffin tin half full with the vegetables.

4. Whisk the egg whites, whole eggs, basil, salt, and pepper in a mixing bowl.

5. Pour the egg mixture slowly into each muffin tin. The egg mixture should fill each tin to the top.

6. Top each cup with a sprinkle of cheese.

7. Bake for 30 minutes or until the muffins have risen and are slightly browned.

8. Serve or keep in the refrigerator for up to 5 days and grab as snacks to go!

NUTRITIONAL INFORMATION: Per 3 Muffins: Calories: 215 kcal; Fat: 7 g; Carbohydrates: 9 g; Protein: 30 g

TUNA TOMATO BITES

Serves: 1

INGREDIENTS

4 sweet cocktail tomatoes (small)

1/2 can water-packed tuna, drained

1/2 tablespoon Dijon mustard

1/2 tablespoon light mayonnaise

1 tablespoon fresh lemon juice

1/4 of a small avocado, diced

1 green onion, diced

2 tablespoons corn kernels (fresh or canned)

1/4 cup 2% cottage cheese

salt and pepper

INSTRUCTIONS

1. Hollow out the tomatoes. Discard the insides or mix them with the tuna.

2. Place the tuna, mustard, mayonnaise, and lemon juice in a bowl and mix well.

3. Add the avocado, green onion, corn, and cottage cheese and fold into tuna mixture.

4. Season with salt and pepper.

5. Stuff into hollowed tomatoes.

NUTRITIONAL INFORMATION: Calories: 220 kcal; Fat: 8 g; Carbohydrates: 12 g; Protein: 23 g

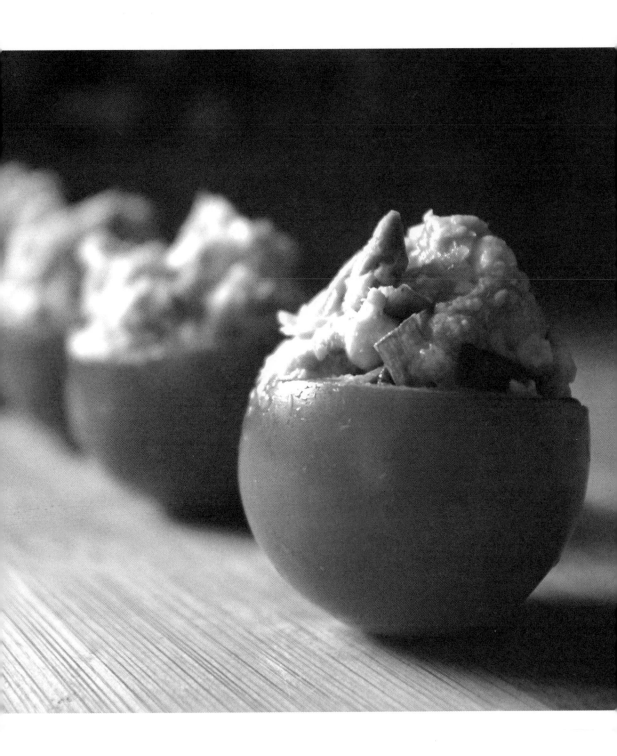

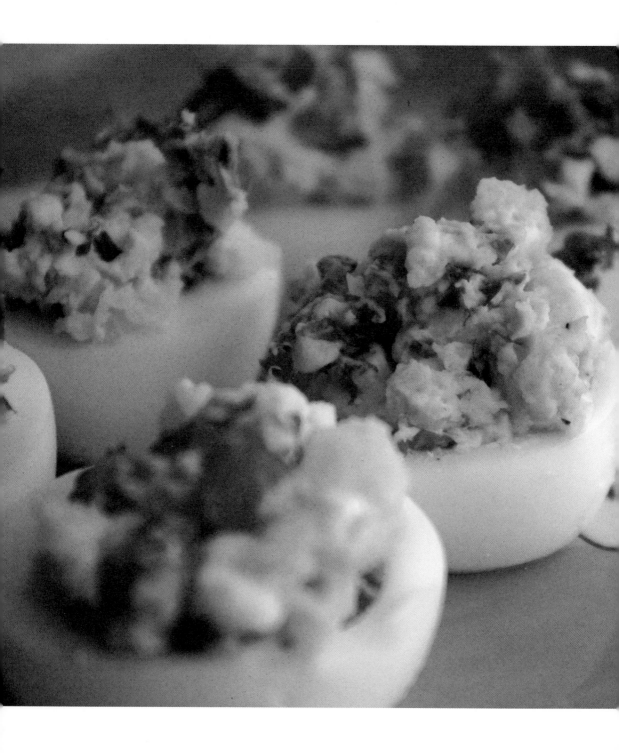

HUMMUS AND KALE DEVILED EGGS

Serves: 1

INGREDIENTS

4 eggs

2 tablespoons prepared hummus (30 calories/tablespoon)

1/4 cup kale, finely chopped

1/4 cup finely diced bell pepper

salt and pepper

INSTRUCTIONS

1. Boil the eggs in boiling water for 8 minutes. Once boiled, remove from the pot and place under cold running water. Peel the eggs and slice in half.

2. Remove the yolks from the eggs and discard 3 of the yolks (or save them for someone else to eat!).

3. In a bowl, combine the remaining 1 yolk and hummus and mash together with a fork.

4. Fold in the kale and bell pepper and season with salt and pepper.

5. Scoop this mixture back into the boiled egg white halves.

NUTRITIONAL INFORMATION: Calories: 205 kcal; Fat: 9 g; Carbohydrates: 8 g; Protein: 24 g

SMOKY CORN AND EDAMAME BEEF CHILI

Serves: 6

INGREDIENTS

1 teaspoon olive oil
1 small onion, diced
1 clove garlic, minced
1¼ pound extra lean ground beef
1 cup sliced mushrooms
1 28-ounce can diced tomatoes
1 8-ounce can tomato paste
1½ cups chicken broth
1 cup frozen corn
1 cup shelled edamame beans
¼ teaspoon salt
   pepper, to taste
1 teaspoon cumin
1 teaspoon paprika
½ teaspoon chili powder
½ teaspoon cayenne powder
1 15-ounce can black beans, rinsed and drained

INSTRUCTIONS

1. In a large pot over medium heat, combine the olive oil, onion, and garlic, and sauté until soft, about 3 minutes.

2. Add the ground beef and mushrooms and cook until browned and the mushrooms are softened, about 7 minutes.

3. Add the diced tomatoes, tomato paste, broth, corn, edamame, salt, pepper, cumin, paprika, chili powder, and cayenne, and bring to a simmer.

4. Reduce the heat to low, add the black beans, and simmer for 20 minutes.

NUTRITIONAL INFORMATION: Serving size: ⅙ of total recipe/ Calories: 370 kcal; Fat: 9 g; Carbohydrates: 38 g; Protein: 36 g

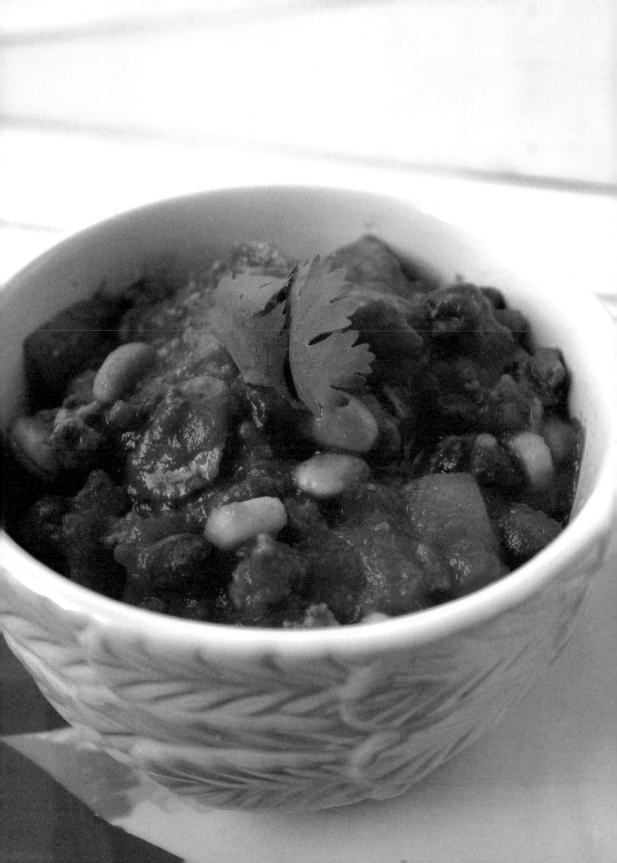

20-MINUTE CHICKEN TORTILLA SOUP

Serves: 6

INGREDIENTS

- 1 teaspoon olive oil
- 1 cup white onion, chopped
- 1 cup bell pepper, chopped
- 2 garlic cloves, minced
- 3/4 teaspoon ground cumin
- 3/4 teaspoon chili powder
- 32 ounces organic chicken broth
- 1 28-ounce can crushed tomatoes
- 15 ounces roasted chicken breast, shredded (rotisserie chicken works great)
- 1/3 cup chopped fresh cilantro
- 1/2 cup coarsely crushed baked organic tortilla chips
- 1/2 cup shredded part-skim mozzarella cheese
- 1 avocado, peeled and diced
- 6 lime wedges

INSTRUCTIONS

1. Heat the oil in a nonstick Dutch oven or large pot on medium-high.

2. Add the onion, bell pepper, and garlic. Cook, stirring often, for 5 minutes or until softened. Stir in the cumin, chili powder, broth, and tomatoes.

3. Bring to a boil. Reduce the heat, and simmer 5 minutes.

4. Add the shredded chicken to the soup and simmer for 3 minutes or until heated through. Stir in the cilantro.

5. Ladle the soup into serving bowls. Top with crushed tortilla chips, cheese, and diced avocado. Serve hot, with a lime wedge on the side.

NUTRITIONAL INFORMATION: Serving size: $1\frac{1}{3}$ cup with 1 tablespoon shredded mozzarella, $\frac{1}{6}$ of an avocado, and 5 tortilla chips/ Calories: 276 kcal; Fat: 10 g; Carbohydrates: 20 g; Protein: 24 g

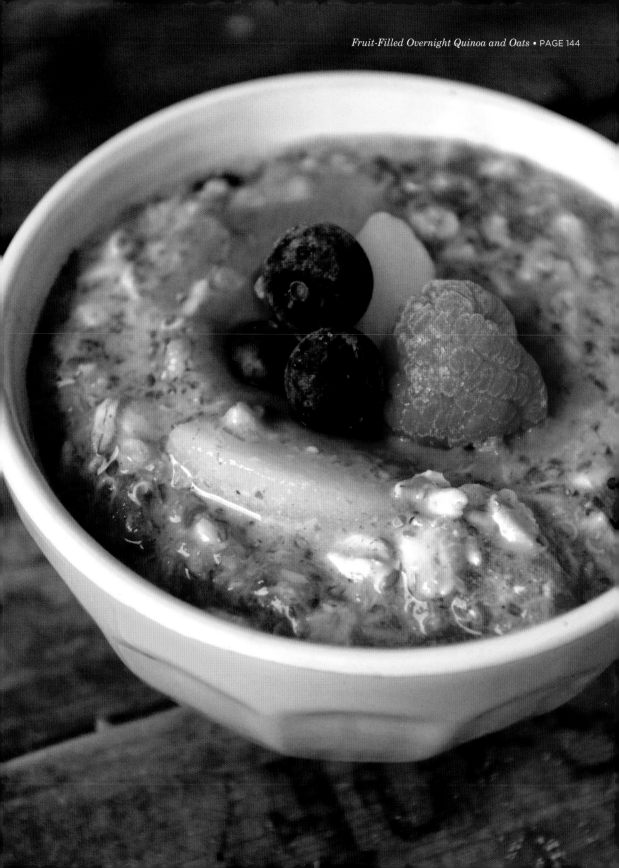

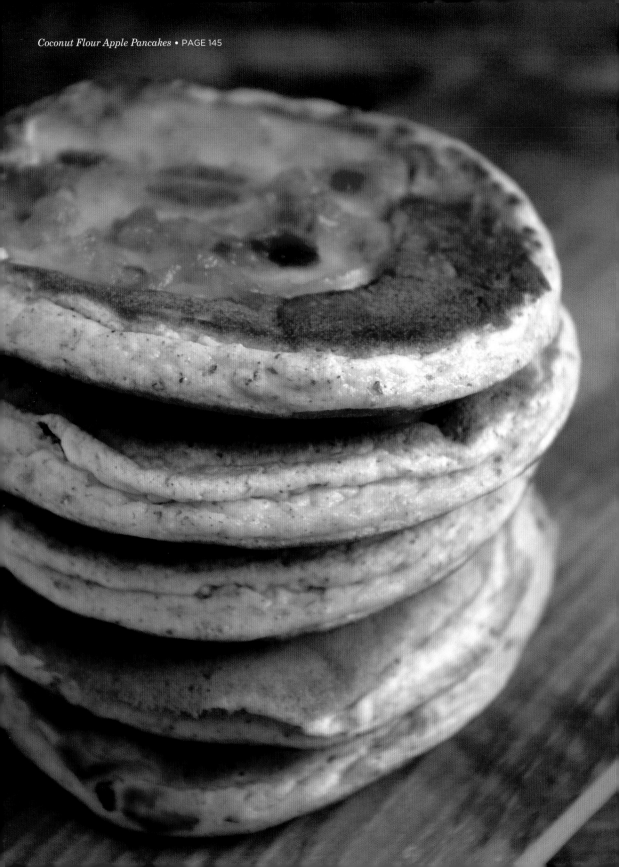

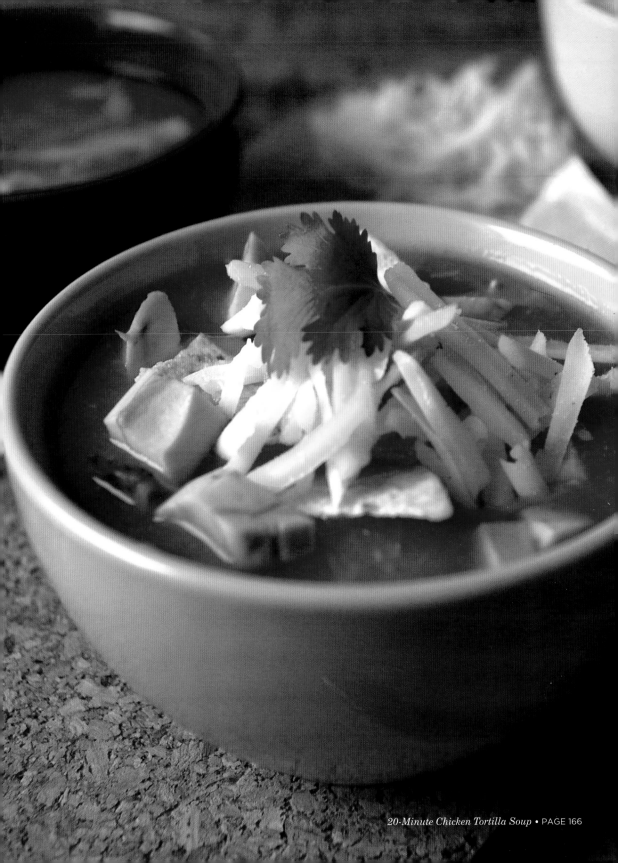

20-Minute Chicken Tortilla Soup • PAGE 166

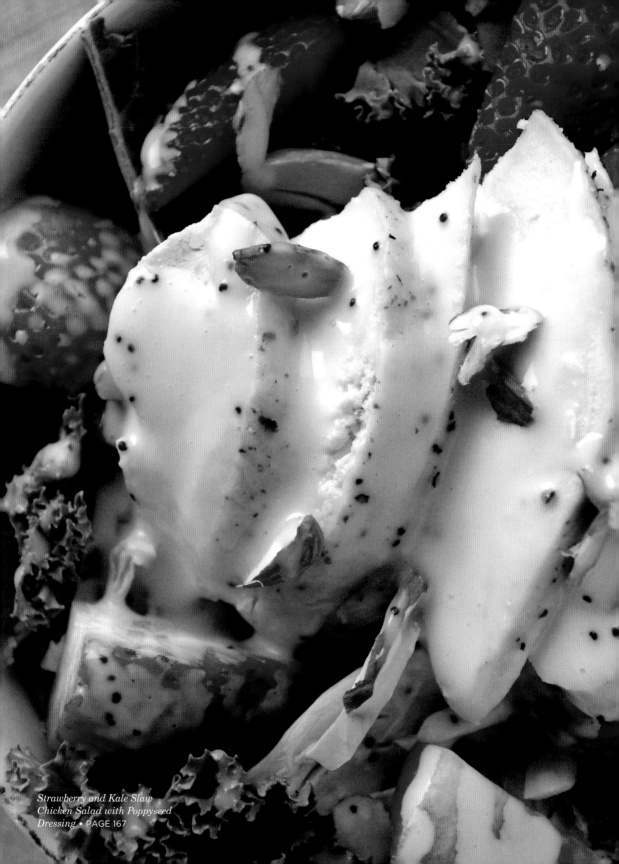

Strawberry and Kale Slaw Chicken Salad with Poppyseed Dressing • PAGE 167

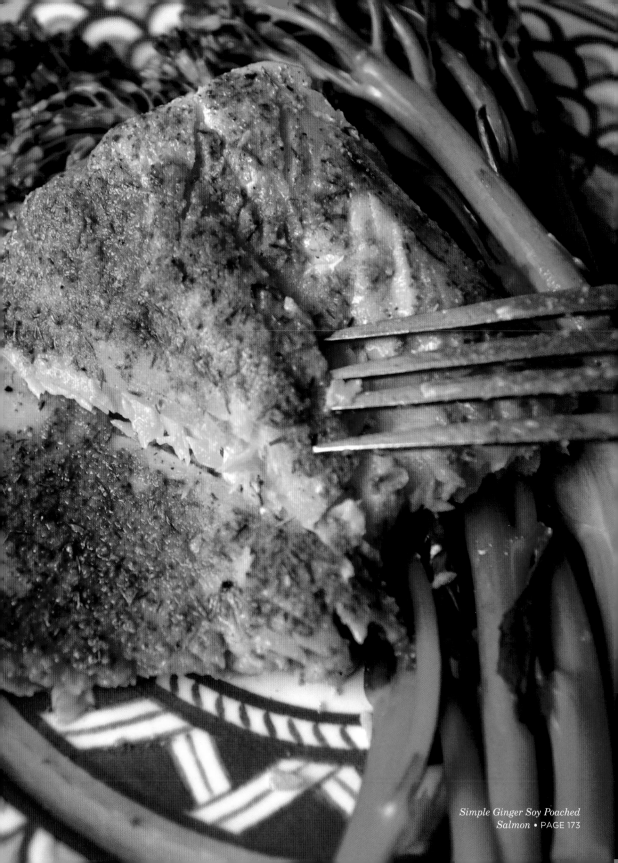

Simple Ginger Soy Poached Salmon • PAGE 173

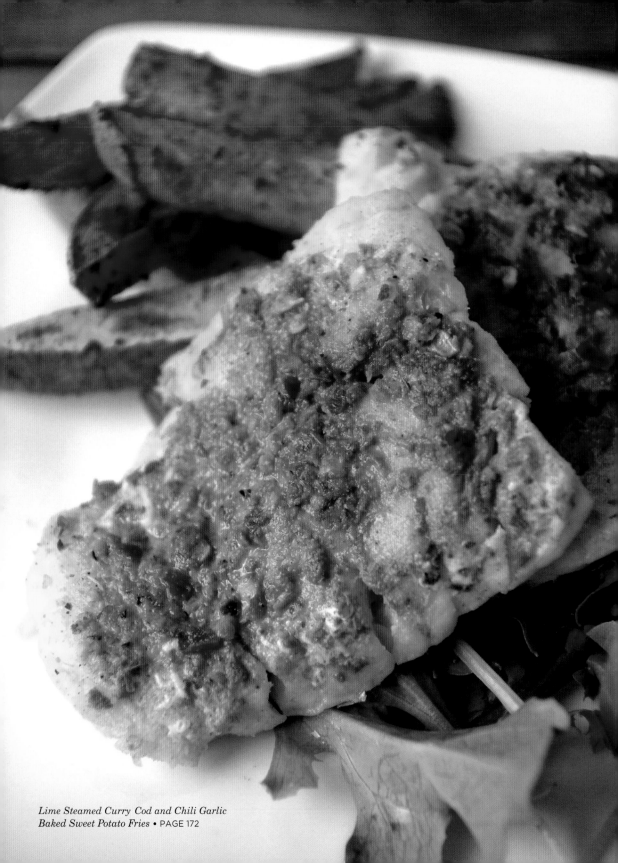

*Lime Steamed Curry Cod and Chili Garlic
Baked Sweet Potato Fries* • PAGE 172

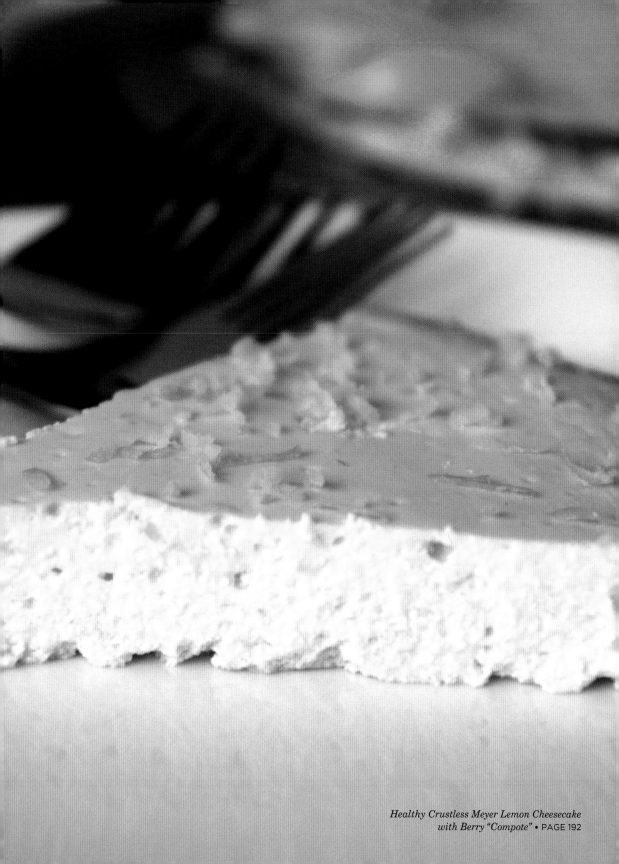

Healthy Crustless Meyer Lemon Cheesecake with Berry "Compote" • PAGE 192

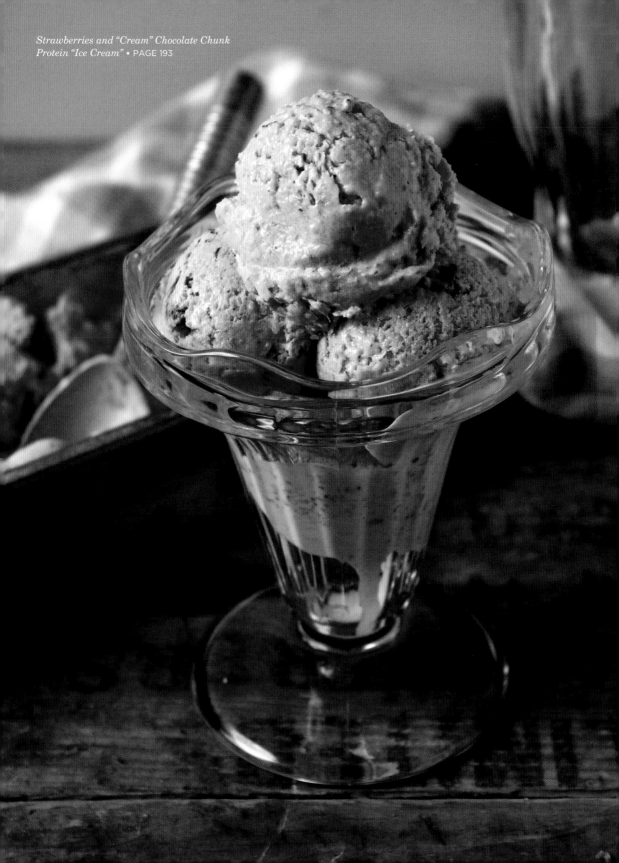

Strawberries and "Cream" Chocolate Chunk
Protein "Ice Cream" • PAGE 193

STRAWBERRY AND KALE SLAW CHICKEN SALAD WITH POPPYSEED DRESSING

Serves: 1

INGREDIENTS

FOR THE DRESSING:
- 1/2 tablespoon light mayonnaise
- 1 teaspoons Dijon mustard
- 1 tablespoon apple cider vinegar
- 1/2 teaspoon lemon juice
- 1 teaspoon agave or honey
- 1/4 teaspoon onion powder
- 1/4 teaspoon garlic powder
- 1/2 teaspoon poppy seeds

FOR THE SALAD:
- 4 ounces chicken breast
- 1/2 cup kale, chopped
- 1/2 cup slaw mix (broccoli slaw, cabbage, carrots mixed)
- 1/4 cup strawberries, sliced

INSTRUCTIONS

1. Whisk together the dressing ingredients and set in the fridge to chill.

2. Bake the chicken breast, cool, and slice.

3. Toss the kale, slaw mix, and strawberries in a bowl.

4. Top with the sliced chicken breast and drizzle the dressing over the salad.

NUTRITIONAL INFORMATION: Calories: 228 kcal; Fat: 6 g; Carbohydrates: 18 g; Protein: 27 g

ASIAN CHICKEN AND SATSUMA SALAD

Serves: 1

INGREDIENTS

DRESSING:

- 1 teaspoon rice wine vinegar
- 1 teaspoon chili garlic sauce
- 1/2 tablespoon low-sodium soy sauce
- 1 teaspoon ground ginger
- 1/2 tablespoon raw honey
- 1 teaspoon sesame oil

SALAD:

- 2 cups romaine lettuce
- 3/4 cup shredded cabbage
- 1/4 cup sugar snap peas, diced
- 1/4 cup sliced red bell pepper
- 1 green onion, sliced
- 1 Satsuma/mandarin orange, peeled and segmented
- 3 ounces plain baked or grilled chicken breast, sliced

INSTRUCTIONS

1. In a small bowl, whisk together the dressing ingredients. Set aside.

2. In a medium bowl, combine the salad ingredients except the chicken.

3. Toss the cooked chicken with half of the dressing and layer it on the salad.

4. Drizzle the remainder of the dressing over the salad.

5. Enjoy!

NUTRITIONAL INFORMATION: Calories: 310 kcal; Fat: 6 g; Carbohydrates: 35 g; Protein: 30 g

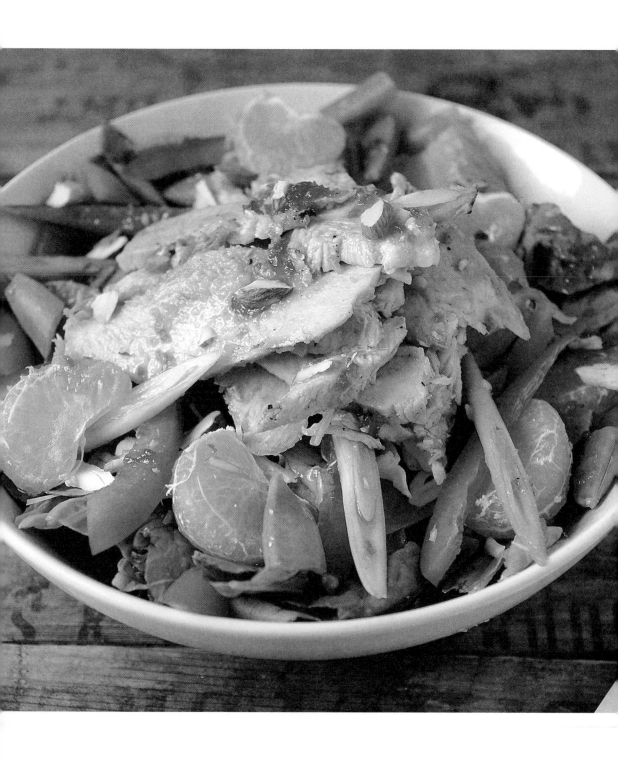

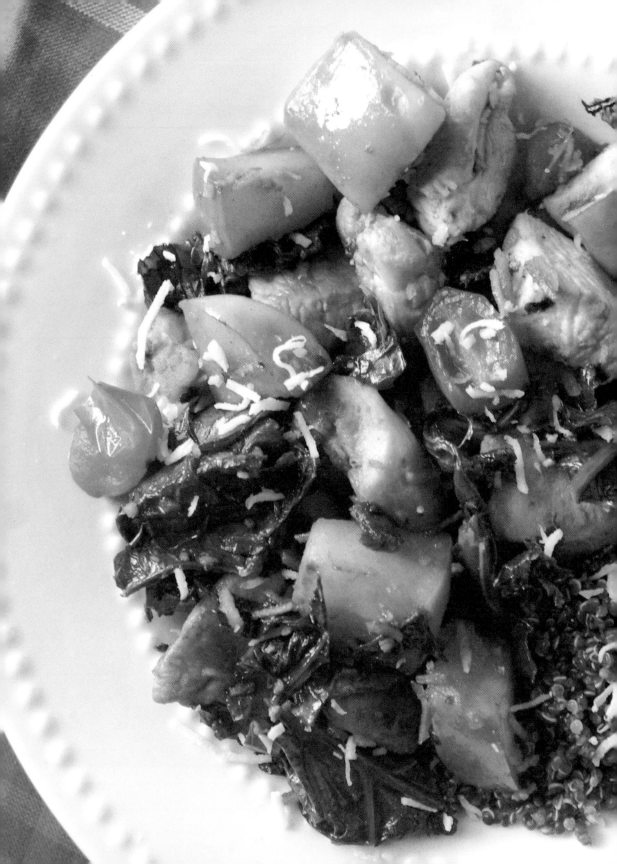

SWEET APPLE, CHICKEN, AND COCONUT SAUTÉ

Serves: 1

INGREDIENTS

4 ounces skinless, boneless chicken breast, diced

1/4 medium gala apple, diced

1/4 teaspoon garlic powder (or 1 clove garlic, minced)

1/4 teaspoon onion powder

salt and pepper

1/4 cup cherry tomatoes, halved

1/2 cup kale, chopped

1 teaspoon pure maple syrup

1/2 tablespoon unsweetened shredded coconut

1 tablespoon water

3/4 cup cooked quinoa

INSTRUCTIONS

1. Heat a large nonstick pan over medium heat and add the diced chicken breast.

2. Add the apple, garlic powder, onion powder, salt, and pepper.

3. Cook for 5–7 minutes. Add the cherry tomatoes, kale, maple syrup, and coconut.

4. Add the water. Simmer the ingredients and wilt the kale.

5. Continue to sauté for 5–7 minutes until chicken is cooked through and browned.

6. Serve with cooked quinoa.

NUTRITIONAL INFORMATION: Calories: 261 kcal; Fat: 5 g; Carbohydrates: 29 g; Protein: 26 g

LIME STEAMED CURRY COD AND CHILI GARLIC BAKED SWEET POTATO FRIES

Serves: 4

INGREDIENTS

FOR THE FRIES:

- 3 medium sweet potatoes, scrubbed and cut into thick strips
- 1 teaspoon garlic powder
- 1 teaspoon chili powder
- 1 teaspoon ground cumin

FOR THE FISH:

- 2 teaspoons dried oregano
- 1 teaspoon chili powder
- 1 teaspoon chili flakes
- 1 teaspoon black pepper
- 2 teaspoons garlic powder
- 2 teaspoons yellow curry powder
- 4 3½-ounce cod fillets
- ⅓ cup fresh lime juice

INSTRUCTIONS

1. Preheat the oven to 400 degrees F. Cut the potatoes and lay them evenly on a baking sheet.

2. Mix the spices for the fries (garlic powder, chili powder, and cumin) in a bowl.

3. Sprinkle the potatoes with the spice mixture and toss until well coated. Bake in the oven for 15 minutes, flip once, and bake for an additional 10 minutes until crispy.

4. Combine all the spices for the fish (oregano, chili powder, chili flakes, pepper, garlic powder, and curry powder) in a bowl.

3. Sprinkle the cod with ½ of the spice mixture and rub gently into the fish. Turn over and repeat for the other side.

4. Pour the lime juice in the bottom of a large skillet and heat to a simmer.

5. Put the fillets in the skillet and cook on medium heat for 4–5 minutes, covered.

6. Remove lid and cook for another 1–2 minutes or until fish easily flakes.

7. Enjoy!

NUTRITIONAL INFORMATION: Serving size: 1 cod fillet and ¼ batch of fries/ Calories: 195 kcal; Fat: 3 g; Carbohydrates: 20 g; Protein: 22 g

SIMPLE GINGER SOY POACHED SALMON

Serves: 4

INGREDIENTS

- 1½ cups brown basmati rice
- 4 cups water, divided use
- ¼ cup low-sodium soy sauce
- 2 tablespoons coconut palm sugar
- ½ teaspoon of your favorite hot sauce or chili pepper flakes
- 2 tablespoons grated ginger
- 4 3.5-ounce fresh salmon fillets
- 4 green onions, thinly sliced
- 20 spears of asparagus

INSTRUCTIONS

1. Cook the rice according to package instructions.

2. Meanwhile, poach the salmon. Match your favorite heavy skillet with a tight-fitting lid.

3. Mix 1 cup of water, the soy sauce, sugar, hot sauce, and ginger together in the skillet.

4. Bring to a vigorous simmer over high heat, then lower to a slow, steady simmer. Nestle the salmon fillets in the mixture and cover the pan. Let simmer for 5 minutes, then gently flip the salmon fillets.

5. Cover and simmer until cooked through, about 4–5 more minutes.

6. Steam the asparagus for 4–5 minutes.

7. Divide the rice and asparagus among four bowls. Position the salmon on each pile of rice and spoon the sauce over the fish evenly. Sprinkle with green onion to garnish.

8. Enjoy!

NUTRITIONAL INFORMATION: Serving size: 1 salmon fillet, with 3/4 cup brown rice, 5 spears asparagus, and sauce/ Calories: 340 kcal; Fat: 7 g; Carbohydrates: 41 g; Protein: 30 g

GRILLED OR BAKED MINI TROPICAL CHICKEN PIZZA

Serves: 1

INGREDIENTS

- 1 thin-style whole grain bun, halved
- ½ tablespoon organic BBQ sauce
- 3 ounces chicken breast, cooked and sliced thin
- 2 tablespoons fresh pineapple, chopped
- 2 tablespoons bell pepper, finely chopped
- 2 tablespoons shredded part-skim mozzarella

INSTRUCTIONS

1. Preheat the grill to low heat, or preheat oven to 325 degrees F.

2. Top each bun half with half the BBQ sauce, chicken breast, pineapple, bell pepper, and shredded cheese.

3. Place on the grill or in the oven for about 10 minutes or until cheese is melted and starting to bubble.

NUTRITIONAL INFORMATION: Calories: 215 kcal; Fat: 4 g; Carbohydrates: 23 g; Protein: 20 g

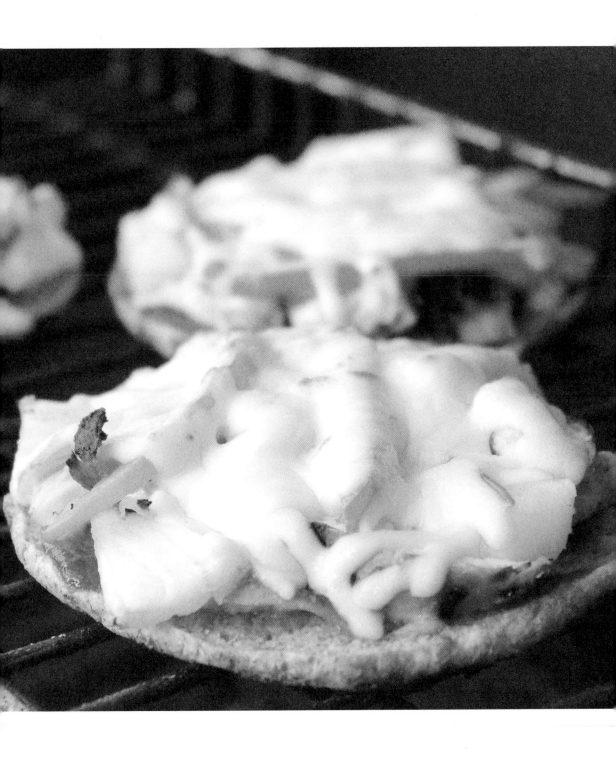

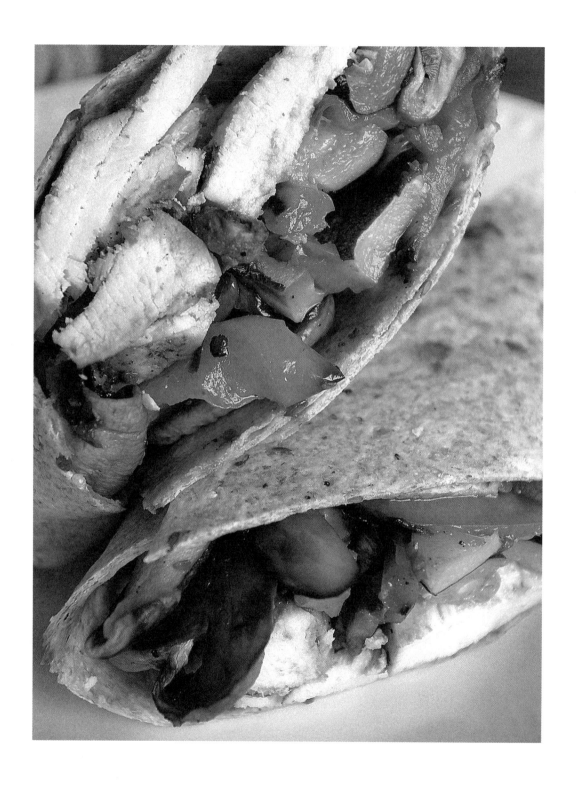

ROASTED VEGETABLE
AND BALSAMIC CHICKEN WRAP

Serves: 2

INGREDIENTS

- 1 cup sliced mushrooms
- 1 zucchini, cut into thick slices
- 1 cup cherry tomatoes, halved
- 1/2 red onion, sliced
- 2 cloves garlic, minced
- 1 bell pepper, sliced
- 1 tablespoon olive oil
- 4 tablespoons aged balsamic vinegar, divided use
- 1 teaspoon Italian seasoning, divided use
- salt and pepper
- 2 4-ounce chicken breasts
- 1 tablespoon fresh basil, minced
- 2 whole grain tortilla wraps

INSTRUCTIONS

1. Preheat the oven to 400 degrees F.

2. Place the mushrooms, zucchini, tomatoes, onion, garlic, and bell pepper on a baking sheet and toss with the olive oil, 2 tablespoons of balsamic vinegar, 1/2 teaspoon Italian seasoning, salt, and pepper.

3. In a bowl, toss the chicken breast with the remaining 2 tablespoons of balsamic vinegar, the remaining 1/2 teaspoon of Italian seasoning, and the basil.

4. Place the chicken on the same or a separate baking sheet.

5. Place everything in the oven and roast for 20 minutes.

6. Remove from oven and let cool slightly.

7. Once cooled, sliced the chicken and assemble the wraps with roasted vegetables!

NUTRITIONAL INFORMATION: Serving size: 1 wrap/ Calories: 346 kcal; Fat: 6 g; Carbohydrates: 40 g; Protein: 32 g

SWEET + SALTY SLOW COOKER CASHEW CHICKEN

Serves: 6

INGREDIENTS

- 2 tablespoons tapioca starch (or arrowroot powder)
- 1/2 teaspoon black pepper
- 1 1/2 pounds raw skinless/boneless chicken breast, diced
- 1 tablespoon coconut oil
- 3 tablespoons gluten-free soy sauce
- 2 tablespoons rice wine vinegar
- 1 tablespoon naturally sweetened ketchup
- 2 tablespoons coconut palm sugar
- 2 minced garlic cloves
- 1 teaspoon minced ginger
- 1/2 cup raw cashews, chopped
- 1 green onion, chopped

INSTRUCTIONS

1. Place the tapioca and pepper in a large plastic bag. Add the chicken pieces and seal; toss to thoroughly coat the meat.

2. Melt the coconut oil in a large nonstick pan. Add the chicken and cook for about 5 minutes until brown on all sides. Remove and add to the slow cooker.

3. Mix the remaining ingredients except for the cashews and green onion in a bowl. Pour the mixture over the chicken and toss to coat. Put the lid on the slow cooker and cook on low for 3–4 hours. Ensure the chicken is fully cooked before moving on to the next step.

4. Stir the cashews into chicken and sauce before serving.

5. Garnish with green onion.

NUTRITIONAL INFORMATION: Serving size: 1/6 of batch/ Calories: 235 kcal; Fat: 7 g; Carbohydrates: 12 g; Protein: 31 g

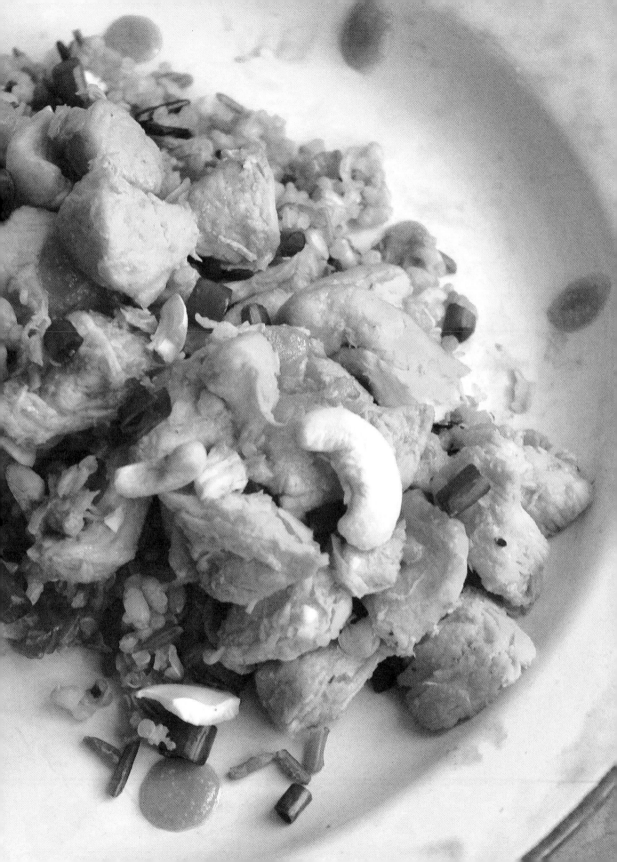

EASY SLOW COOKER PULLED CHICKEN

Serves: 6

INGREDIENTS

- 1/2 onion, chopped
- 1 pound boneless skinless chicken breasts
- juice of 1/2 lime
- 1 28-ounce can crushed tomatoes
- 1 tablespoon cumin
- 2 teaspoon chili powder
- 1 teaspoon cayenne
- 2 teaspoon garlic powder
- 1 teaspoon onion powder

INSTRUCTIONS

1. Place the onion in the bottom of the slow cooker. Add the chicken, and pour the lime juice and crushed tomatoes on top.

2. Add the remaining ingredients, and mix everything to combine.

3. Cook on low for 6 hours.

4. With two forks, shred the chicken breasts and mix well.

NUTRITIONAL INFORMATION: Serving size: 1/6 of the batch/ Calories: 212 kcal; Fat: 4 g; Carbohydrates: 9 g; Protein: 33 g

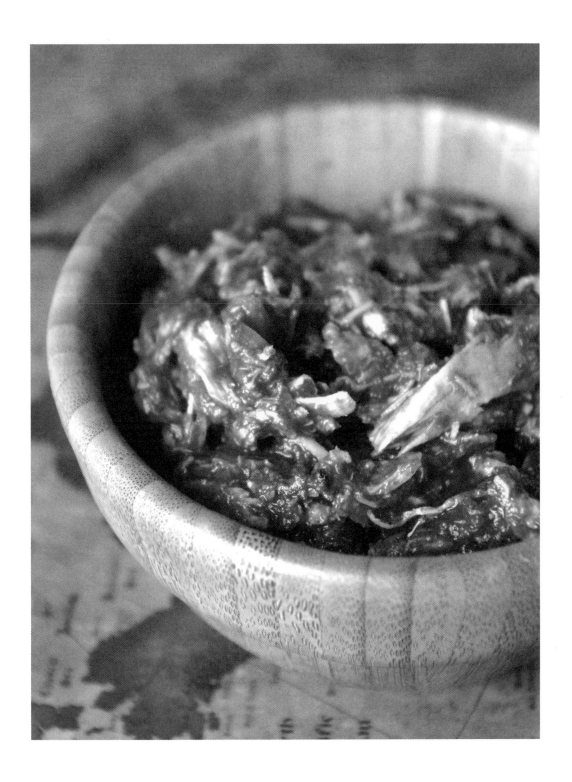

SWEET POTATO, KALE, AND TURKEY CHILI

Serves: 4

INGREDIENTS

- 1 pound extra lean ground turkey
- ½ teaspoon salt
- ½ teaspoon cumin
- ½ cup onion, chopped
- 3 cloves garlic, crushed
- 1½ cups canned diced tomatoes
- 1 medium sweet potato, peeled and diced into small cubes (½ pound)
- 1½ cups tomato sauce
- ¾ cup water
- ¼ teaspoon chili powder
- ¼ teaspoon paprika
- 1 cup chopped kale
- fresh cilantro, for garnish

INSTRUCTIONS

1. In a large skillet, brown the turkey over medium-high heat, breaking it up as it cooks into smaller pieces. Season with salt and cumin.

2. When the meat is browned and cooked through, add the onion and garlic and cook for 3 minutes over medium heat. Add the diced tomatoes, sweet potato, tomato sauce, water, chili powder, and paprika.

3. Cover and simmer over medium-low heat until the potatoes are soft and cooked through, about 20 minutes, stirring occasionally. Add ¼ cup more water if needed.

4. Add the chopped kale, and stir until the kale is wilted.

5. Top with a sprig of cilantro and serve.

NUTRITIONAL INFORMATION: Serving size: ¼ recipe/
Calories: 245 kcal; Fat: 7 g; Carbohydrates: 22 g; Protein: 27 g

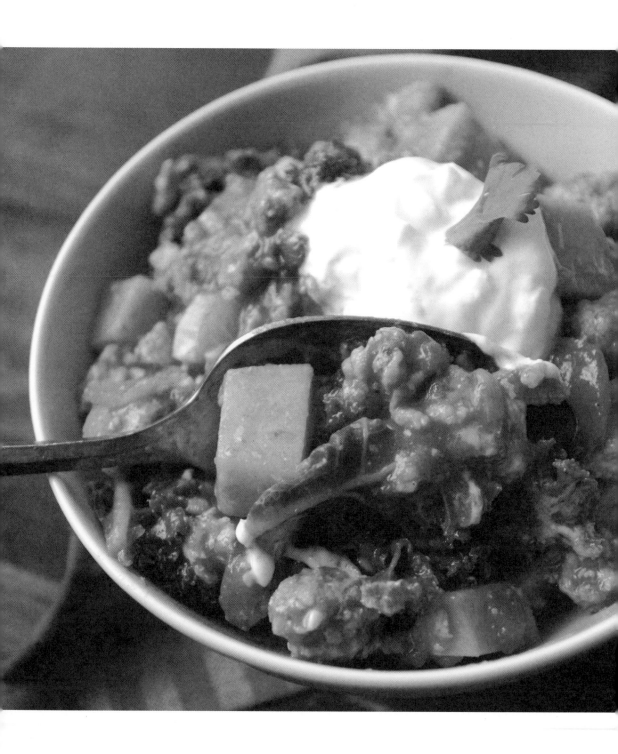

TURKEY, APPLE BUTTER, AND ARUGULA GRILLED CHEESE

Serves: 1

INGREDIENTS

cooking spray

1 tablespoon apple butter

2 slices whole grain bread

1 slice organic cheddar cheese (approximately 1 ounce)

4 ounces cooked turkey breast filet, thinly sliced

1/4 cup arugula

INSTRUCTIONS

1. Heat a nonstick pan over medium heat, and apply a small amount of cooking spray.

2. Spread the apple butter over the surface of each piece of bread. Top one slice with half of the cheese, the turkey breast, then the other half of the cheese, and arugula.

3. Place the other piece of bread apple butter side down to make a sandwich. Press firmly.

4. Cook in the pan for 2 minutes on each side, or until the bread is browned and the cheese is melted.

NUTRITIONAL INFORMATION: Calories: 300 kcal; Fat: 4 g; Carbohydrates: 28 g; Protein: 36 g

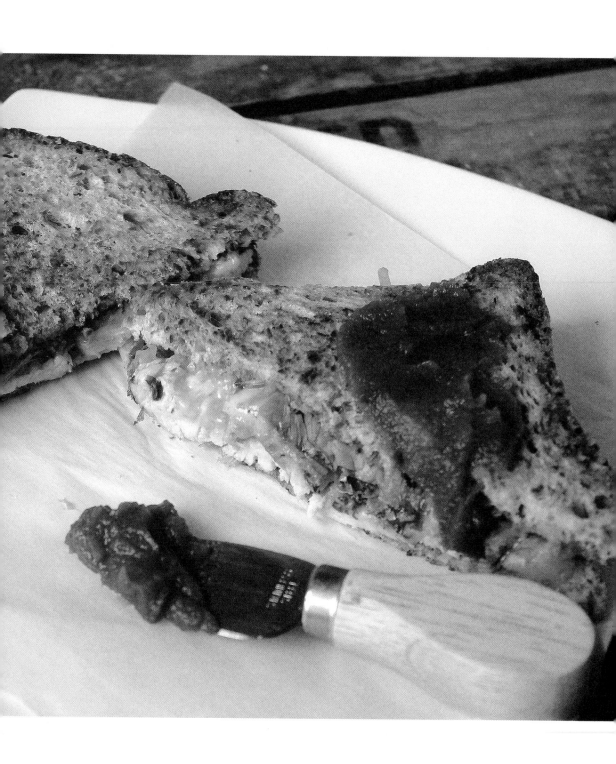

ORANGE "CREAMSICLE" SMOOTHIE

Serves: 1

INGREDIENTS

- 1 large banana, cut into chunks and frozen
- 1 small navel orange, peeled and separated, then frozen
- 1 scoop no additives, naturally sweetened whey isolate or whey concentrate (or add cocoa powder to vanilla flavor)
- 1 teaspoon turmeric (optional, solely for a color boost)
- 1/4 teaspoon pure orange extract (optional)
- 4 large ice cubes

INSTRUCTIONS

1. Cut and freeze the banana and orange ahead of time.

2. Place the frozen banana, orange, whey, turmeric, extract, and ice in a blender and blend until a smooth thick consistency is reached.

NUTRITIONAL INFORMATION: Calories: 275 kcal; Fat: 2 g; Carbohydrates: 42 g; Protein: 27 g

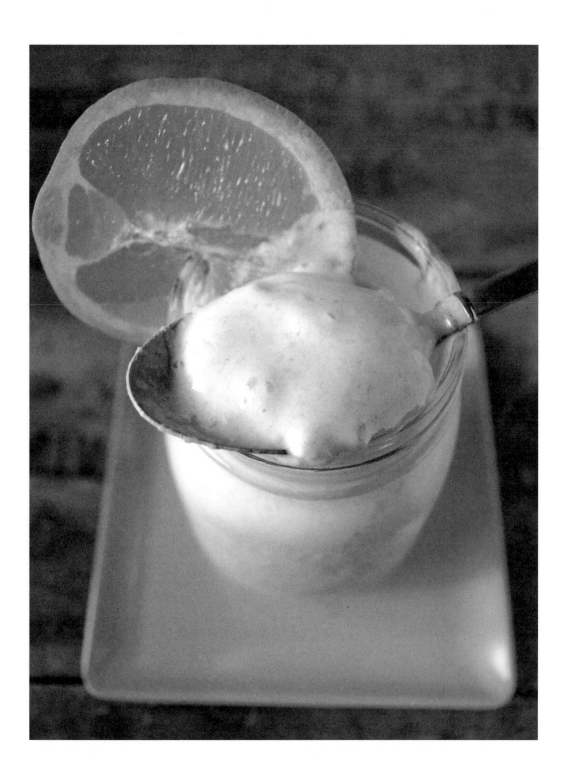

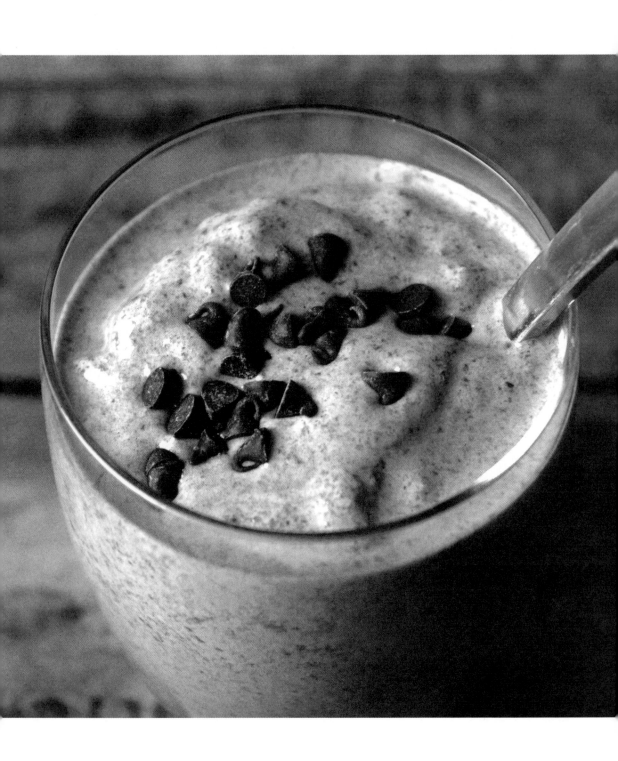

MINT CHOCOLATE
GREEN PROTEIN SMOOTHIE

Serves: 1

INGREDIENTS

- 1 scoop no-additives, naturally sweetened chocolate whey isolate or whey concentrate (add 1 teaspoon cocoa powder if you do not have chocolate-flavored whey)
- 1 tablespoon ground flaxseed
- 1 medium banana (peeled, cut into sections, and frozen)
- ½ cup fresh spinach (or frozen)
- ¼ teaspoon pure peppermint extract
- stevia to taste
- 3–4 ice cubes
- ¼ cup unsweetened almond milk
- 1 tablespoon 70% dark chocolate chips

INSTRUCTIONS

1. Blend all ingredients except the chocolate chips. The mixture will be very thick, so make sure you have a good blender! If you prefer a thinner consistency, add some water.

2. Garnish with the dark chocolate chips.

NUTRITIONAL INFORMATION: Calories: 360 kcal; Fat: 8 g; Carbohydrates: 39 g; Protein: 37 g

FIG AND CHOCOLATE
FROZEN PROTEIN FUDGE

Serves: 8

INGREDIENTS

1¼ cup dried figs

1¾ cup hot water

1 tablespoon pure vanilla

⅓ cup natural almond butter

⅓ cup raw hemp seeds

chocolate stevia and/or cocoa powder (to your taste— makes it "chocolaty")

INSTRUCTIONS

1. Place the figs in a bowl, cover with hot water, and soak for about 1 hour until soft. Drain, and reserve the liquid.

2. In a blender (or food processor), blend the figs and vanilla until smooth, slowly adding the reserved water as needed to form a creamy consistency.

3. Transfer the fig mixture to a large bowl, add the almond butter and hemp seeds, and stir to combine.

4. Gradually add the dry protein mixture to the wet fig mixture, and stir well. Add chocolate stevia and/ or cocoa powder to your taste.

5. Press or smooth evenly into an 8×8 baking pan and freeze until firm (about 3 hours).

6. Cut into 8 bars and serve.

NUTRITIONAL INFORMATION: Serving size: 1 bar/ Calories: 135 kcal; Fat: 7 g; Carbohydrates: 16 g; Protein: 5 g

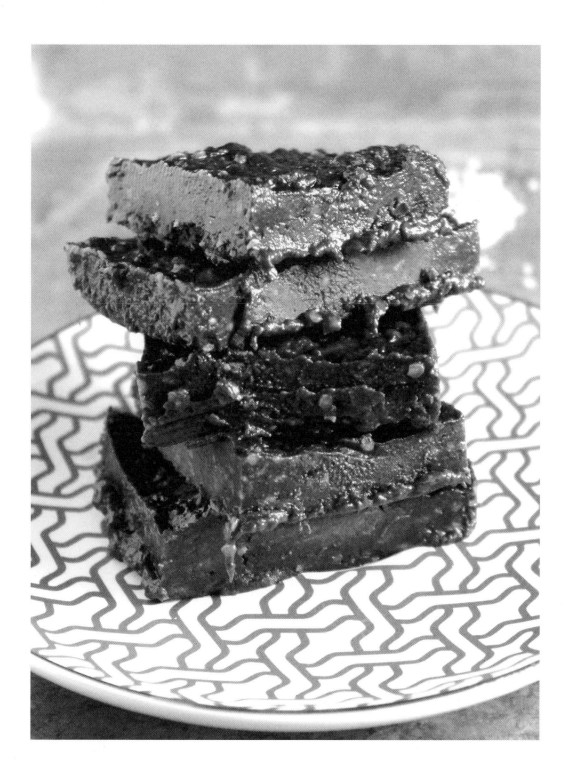

HEALTHY CRUSTLESS MEYER LEMON CHEESECAKE WITH BERRY "COMPOTE"

Serves: 3

INGREDIENTS

- 1/2 cup dry curd cottage cheese
- 2/3 cup plain 0% Greek yogurt
- zest of 1 Meyer lemon, divided use
- juice of 1 whole Meyer lemon
- 2 teaspoons pure vanilla extract
- 1/2 teaspoon pure lemon extract (optional, for extra lemony flavor)
- 2 whole eggs
- 1 egg white
- 3 tablespoons baking stevia (or 5 packets stevia)
- 1 tablespoon pure honey
- 1/4 teaspoon salt
- 1/2 cup berries of choice

INSTRUCTIONS

1. Preheat the oven to 350 degrees F.

2. In a blender or food processor, pulse the cottage cheese, yogurt, half of the lemon zest, the lemon juice, vanilla, lemon extract, eggs, egg white, stevia, honey, and salt until as smooth as possible.

3. Line the bottom of a lightly greased cake pan with parchment paper to prevent sticking. Pour the mixture into the pan.

4. Bake for 45 minutes, remove from the oven, and cool to room temperature on a cooling rack.

5. When the cake is cool, heat the berries for 20 seconds in the microwave and mash them together with the remaining lemon zest with a fork to make a berry "compote" for the cheesecake.

6. Cut the entire cake into three large slices—1 slice plus 1/3 of the berry sauce is 1 serving.

NUTRITIONAL INFORMATION: Serving size: 1/ Calories: 230 kcal; Fat: 4 g; Carbohydrates: 10 g; Protein: 32 g

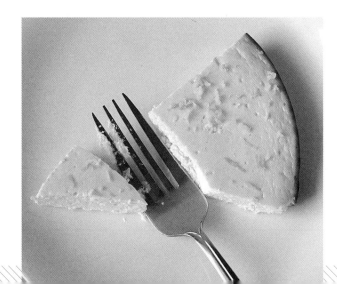

STRAWBERRIES AND "CREAM" CHOCOLATE CHUNK PROTEIN "ICE CREAM"

Serves: 1

INGREDIENTS

- ⅓ banana
- ¾ cup frozen strawberries
- 1 scoop no-additives, naturally sweetened whey isolate or whey concentrate
- 1–2 tablespoons unsweetened almond milk
- ⅓ ounce 70% dark chocolate, cut into chunks

INSTRUCTIONS

1. Cut the banana into pieces and place in the freezer for 3 hours.

2. Once the banana pieces are frozen, blend them in a food processor with the strawberries and whey until it is the consistency of soft-serve ice cream. You may need to add in 1–2 tablespoons of almond milk if the mixture is too thick.

3. Fold in the chocolate chunks, transfer the ice cream to a container, and freeze until it reaches the desired consistency (1 hour or so for typical ice cream texture).

NUTRITIONAL INFORMATION: Calories: 50 kcal; Fat: 8 g; Carbohydrates: 23 g; Protein: 27 g

HEALTHY ALMOND PISTACHIO FROZEN YOGURT

Serves: 1

INGREDIENTS

- 1 cup 0% fat plain Greek yogurt
- 1 medium banana, sliced into chunks and frozen
- 1/2 cup raw spinach
- 1 ounce ripe avocado
- 2 packets stevia (or 10 drops of liquid stevia)
- 1/4 teaspoon pure almond extract
- 2 ice cubes
- 1 tablespoon pistachios, shelled

INSTRUCTIONS

1. In a blender or food processor, blend together the yogurt, frozen banana, spinach, avocado, stevia, almond extract, and ice.

2. You may need to pulse and blend a few times while scraping the sides. (If you have an ice cream maker, you can pour this mixture into your machine and finish according to the manufacturer's instructions.)

3. Once well blended, pour the mixture into a bowl and sprinkle with pistachios.

4. Freeze for 2–3 hours until firm enough to scoop with a spoon like ice cream.

NUTRITIONAL INFORMATION: Calories: 290 kcal; Fat: 5 g; Carbohydrates: 38 g; Protein: 27 g

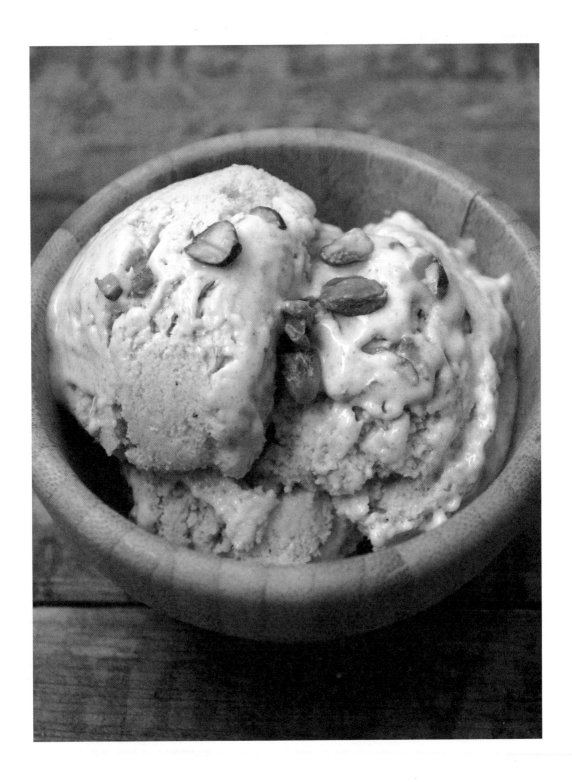

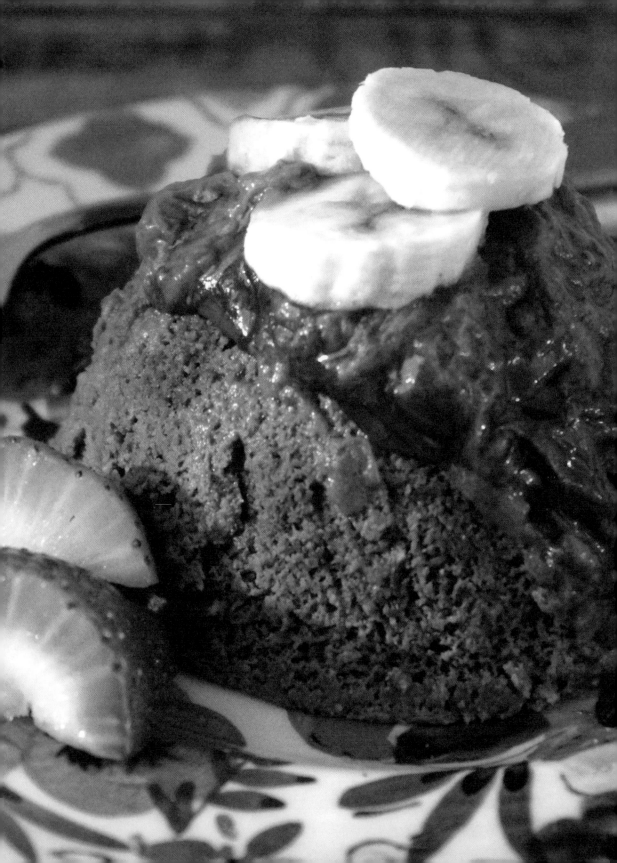

1-MINUTE BANANA SPLIT MUG CAKE

Serves: 1

INGREDIENTS

- 1 tablespoon coconut flour
- 3 tablespoons no-additives, naturally sweetened whey isolate or whey concentrate
- 1 tablespoon peanut flour (PB2 brand, if possible)
- 2 teaspoons ground flaxseed
- 1/2 teaspoon baking powder
- stevia to taste (or 5–10 drops liquid stevia)
- 1 teaspoon raw cocoa powder
- 1/4 cup mashed banana
- 2 tablespoons egg whites (1 egg white)
- 3 tablespoons unsweetened almond milk
- 1/2 tablespoon natural peanut butter for topping
- 1 sliced strawberry for topping

INSTRUCTIONS

1. In a large mug combine the coconut flour, whey, peanut flour, flaxseed, baking powder, stevia (if using liquid stevia, mix it into the wet ingredients in step 2 instead), and cocoa powder. Mix well to eliminate clumps.

2. In a small bowl, combine the banana, egg whites, and almond milk, and stir well (this might be a little clumpy still because of the banana, and that's okay!).

3. Mix the wet mixture into the dry mixture and stir well.

4. Cover the mug with plastic wrap or another cover of choice and microwave on high for 1 minute.

5. Remove mug from microwave and either eat right out of the mug or tip over onto a plate.

6. Top with peanut butter and the strawberry.

NUTRITIONAL INFORMATION: Calories: 260 kcal; Fat: 11 g; Carbohydrates: 21 g; Protein: 26 g

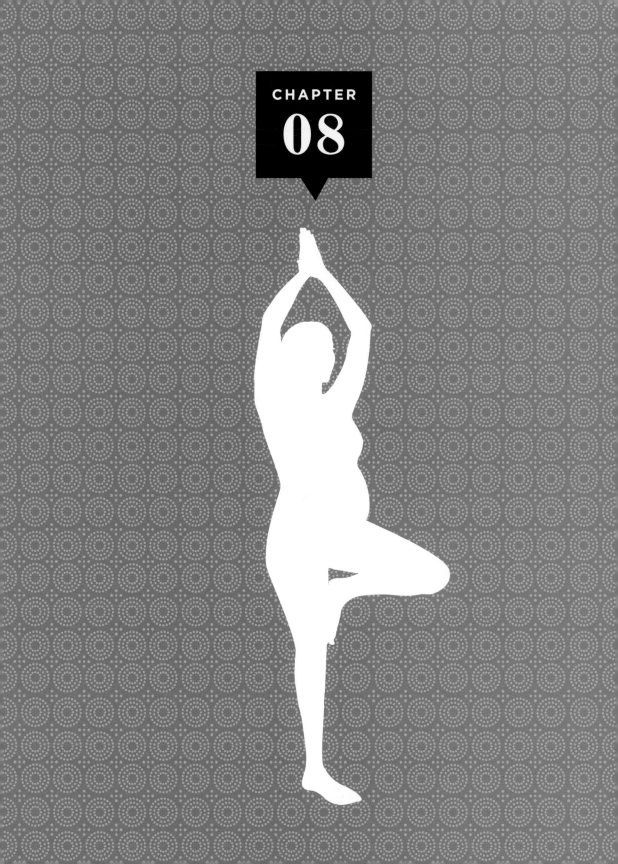

YOUR FIT PREGNANCY EXERCISE

DESCRIPTIONS AND DEMONSTRATIONS

→ A growing belly and changing body needs exercises selected just for you! These moves will help you keep moving for nine months and beyond.

Model: Erica Willick (author)

21s This move has three parts, and each part has 7 repetitions for a total of 21 repetitions. Start by holding a barbell, standing with your feet shoulder width apart and letting your arms hang at your sides.

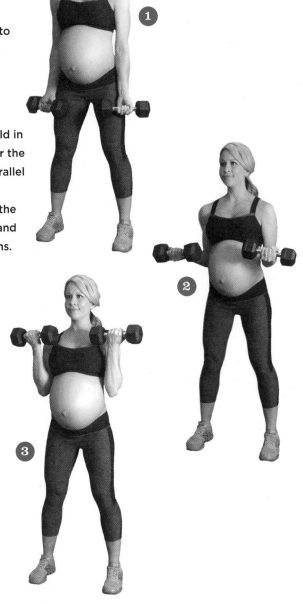

PART 1
Curl the barbell upward until your forearms are parallel with the ground (when you reach halfway up/the midpoint), then lower the weight to the initial position and repeat this motion for 7 repetitions.

PART 2
Without resting, curl the weight completely to the top as you would in a traditional bicep curl, then lower the weight until your forearms are parallel with the ground (when you reach halfway up/midpoint), then raise the weight to the top initial position and repeat this motion for 7 repetitions.

PART 3
Once again without resting, curl the weight the entire range of motion for 7 repetitions.

Alternating Dumbbell Curl

Stand with feet shoulder width apart, holding two dumbbells in front of you. Your low back should be in, and your chest should be high.

1 Hold each dumbbell against the front of you thighs, palms facing away from your thighs.

2 Keeping your elbows close to your body, curl the right dumbbell to your chest without swinging.

3 Slowly lower the dumbbell back to your thighs and then repeat the motion on your left side to complete 1 repetition.

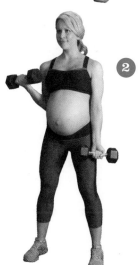

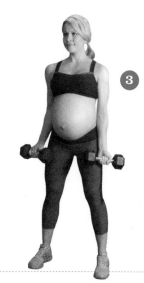

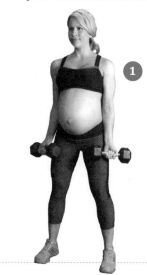

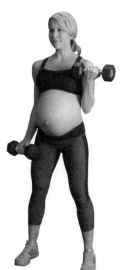

Arnold Press
Sit on the end of an exercise bench with your feet flat on the floor.

1 Hold two dumbbells in front of your face with your palms facing you and elbows bent.

2 Move your hands apart while rotating the palms of your hands until they are facing forward. Keep your hands above shoulder height.

3 Next, press your hands overhead until the dumbbells touch.

4 Reverse the motion to complete 1 repetition.

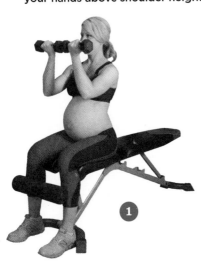

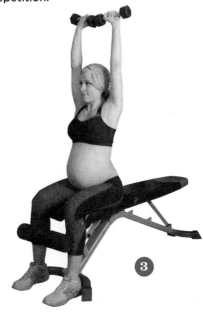

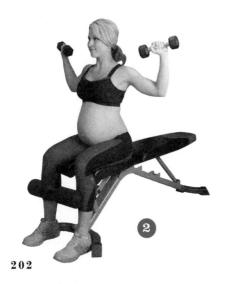

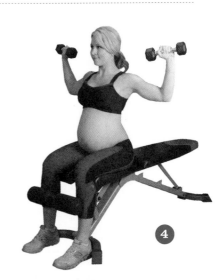

Barbell Curl
Stand with feet shoulder width apart, gripping a barbell in front of you. Your lower back should be in, and your chest should be high.

1 Hold the barbell with your palms facing outward, hands just outside your thighs.

2 Keeping your elbows close to your body, curl the barbells to your chest. No swinging.

3 Slowly lower the barbells back to your thighs to complete 1 repetition.

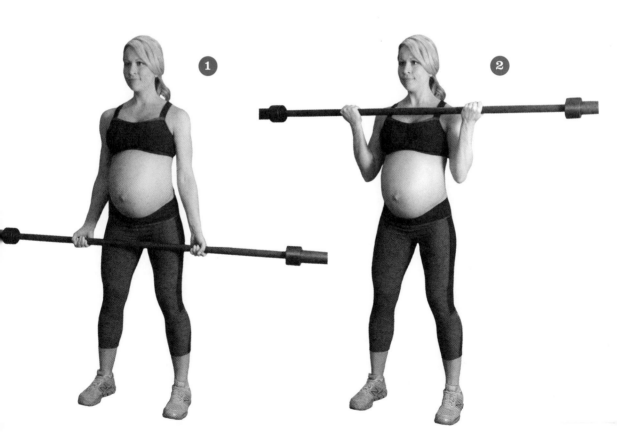

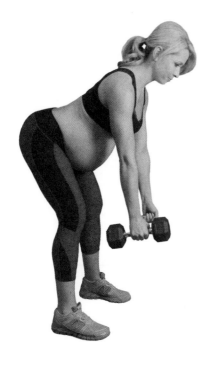
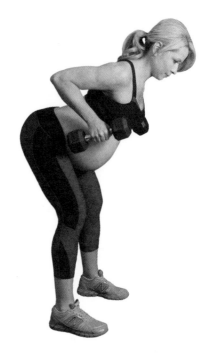

Bent-over Standing Row

Gripping two dumbbells, stand with your feet slightly wider than shoulder width (far enough apart to accommodate your baby belly).

1 Hinging at the hips, bend forward. Be sure to keep your low back naturally tucked in and chest high. Your neck stays in alignment with your spine.

2 Palms of hands facing each other.

3 Slowly pull the dumbbells to your chest, pause for one second, then lower the dumbells. Repeat this pull-up and lower-down motion for the prescribed number of reps.

Bird Dog Start on your hands and knees, ensuring that your wrists are underneath your shoulders and your fingers are pointing forward.

1 Engage your core and keep your spine in neutral position. The goal is to move the opposite arm and leg simultaneously; however, start the first few by slowly lengthening your left leg, then raising and straightening your right arm until you get comfortable with the movement. Avoid rotating your hip and keep your face down so your spine is in alignment.

2 Switch to the opposite side (right leg/left arm) and continue back and forth for the prescribed number of repetitions.

3 If you feel you are straining through your core or your core is not staying engaged, stop the exercise.

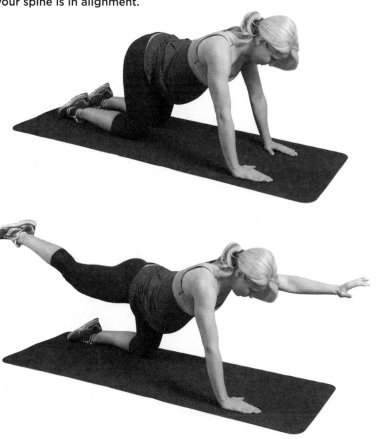

BOSU Preggo "Burpee" This is a low-impact movement and a modified version of the traditional Burpee. Using the BOSU balance trainer gives your shoulders a workout in the process! The traditional jump back in this move should be a small and gentle hop. As your belly grows, remove the push-up portion of this move.

1 Squat down and place your hands on the BOSU (round side down), and hop your feet back so that you are in the push-up position.

2 Lower your chest to the flat side of the BOSU and press back up to complete the push-up.

3 While continuing to hold the BOSU, stand up, then press the BOSU overhead.

4 Reverse the motion to complete 1 repetition.

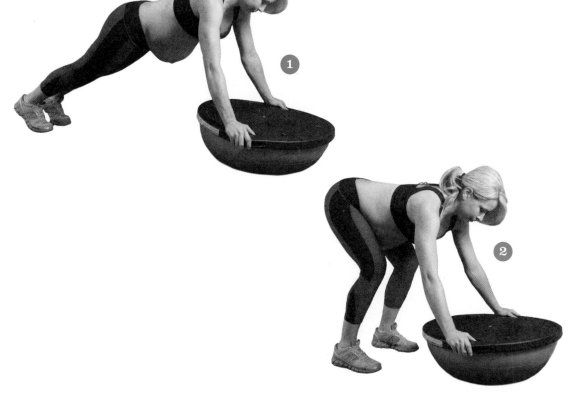

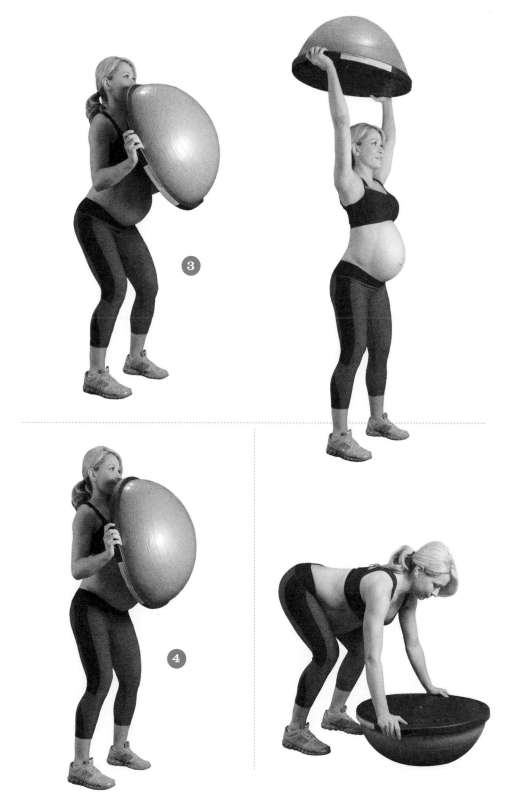

Cable Front Raise
Set the cable machine to the low setting and attach the standard handle. Grasp the handle in your left hand, and stand facing away from the cable machine.

1 Start with your left hand by your left side.

2 Extend your left arm forward until your hand is level with your shoulder. Do not lock your elbow.

3 Reverse the motion to complete 1 repetition.

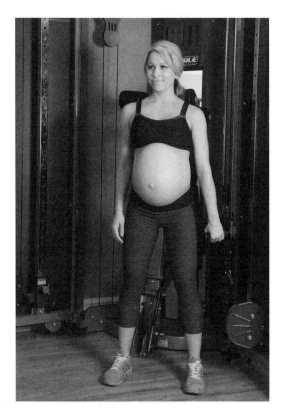
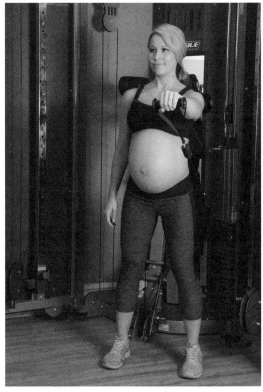

Cable Overhead Rope Extension
Set the cable machine to the high setting and attach the rope. Face away from the cable machine and grasp the rope overhead. Your right foot is slightly ahead of your left foot and your knees are slightly bent.

1 To start, your elbows are bent with your arms close to your head.

2 Your elbows stay beside your head as you extend your hands upward, pressing through your triceps.

3 Reverse the motion to complete 1 repetition.

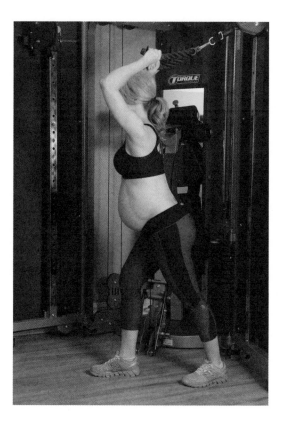
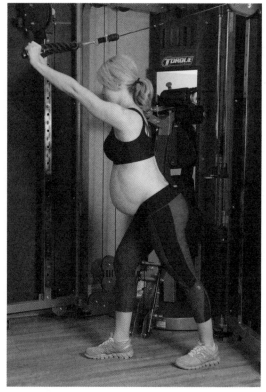

Cable Pull-through

Start by standing a few feet in front of a low cable pulley with a rope or handle attached. Face away from the machine, straddling the cable, with your feet wider than shoulder width apart.

1 Keeping your knees bent, reach through your legs as far as possible, bending at the hips.

2 Keep your arms straight as you extend through your hips to stand up straight. The motion is through your hips to target your legs, not your arms/shoulders. Ensure that you keep your low back naturally tucked in and chest high.

3 The alternate exercise is a seated hamstring curl, which is found at most gyms.

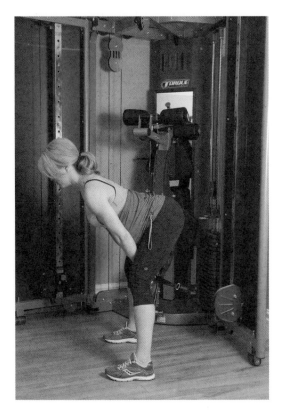

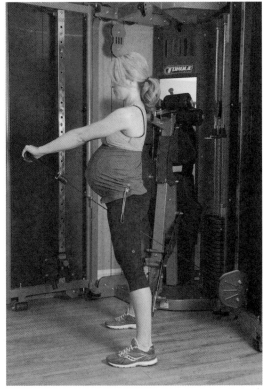

Cable Woodchop

Move the cable machine to the highest pulley position and connect a standard handle. With your side to the cable machine, grab the handle with both hands and take one step away from the machine. Feet are shoulder width apart.

1 In one motion, pull the handle down and across your body while rotating your torso. Pivot your back foot and bend your knee. Keep your arms and back straight and core tight throughout the movement.

2 Return to starting position in a slow and controlled manner to complete 1 repetition.

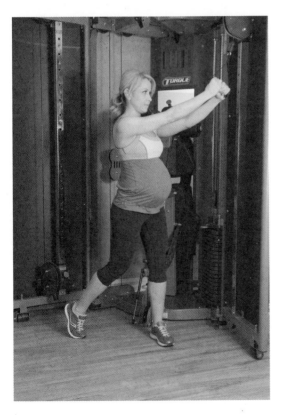
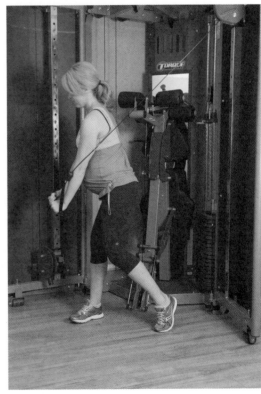

Calf Raises (Toes in)

Stand on a step with your heels hanging off the edge of the step.

Point your toes inward, slowly stretch your heels down to the bottom of the motion, then push up through your toes to the top. Ensure you get full range of motion.

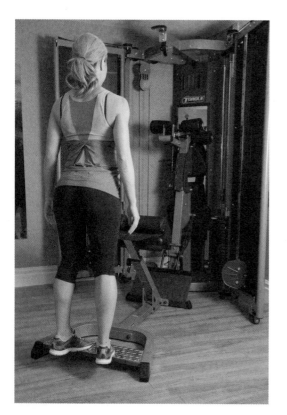

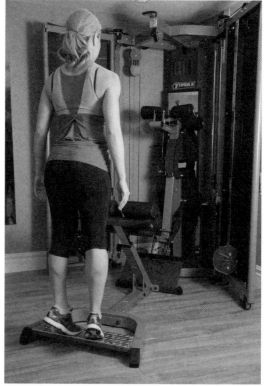

Calf Raises (Toes out)
Stand on a step with your heels hanging off the edge of the step.

Point your toes outward, slowly stretch your heels down to the bottom of the motion, then push up through your toes to the top. Ensure you get full range of motion.

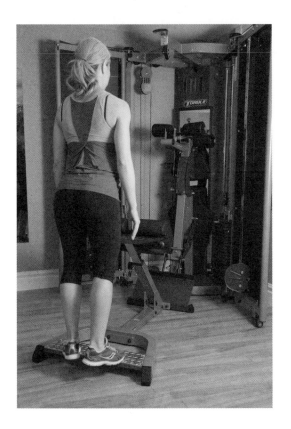
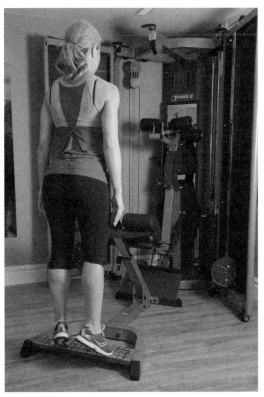

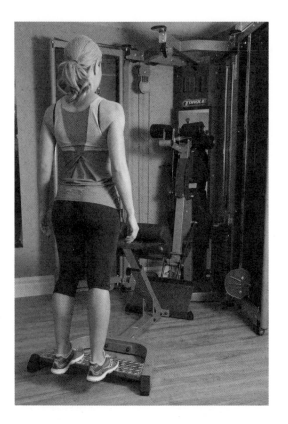 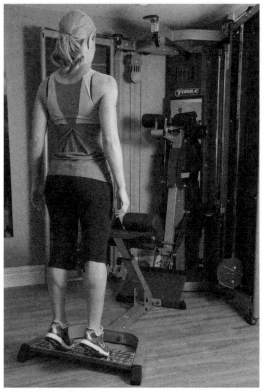

Calf Raises (Toes Straight)

Stand on a step with your heels hanging off the edge of the step.

Point your toes forward, slowly stretch your heels down to the bottom of the motion, then push up through your toes to the top. Ensure you get full range of motion.

Concentration Curl Sit on a flat bench and spread your legs wide, dumbbell in your right hand.

1 Lean forward, keeping your back straight. Place your right elbow on the inside of your right leg just above your knee.

2 Curl the dumbbell until it touches your bicep. Slowly reverse the movement to complete 1 repetition.

3 Once the right side repetitions are complete, switch sides to finish the set.

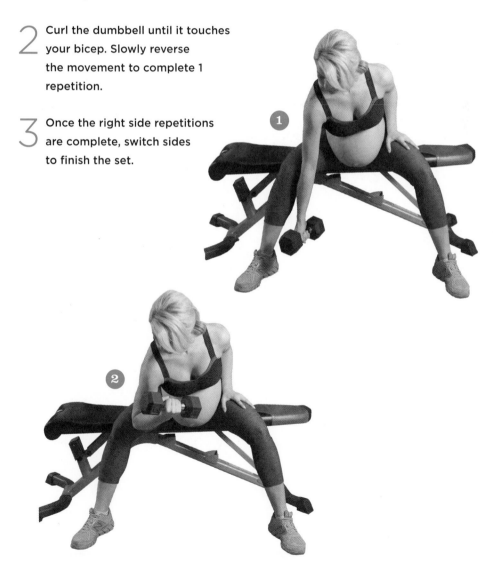

Cross-overs

Set the dual cable system to the high setting with the standard handles attached on each pulley. Face away from the cable machine and grasp a handle in each hand. Feet are shoulder width apart.

1 Pull the cables together, keeping a slight bend in your elbows and focusing on squeezing with your chest.

2 Slowly reverse the movement to complete 1 repetition.

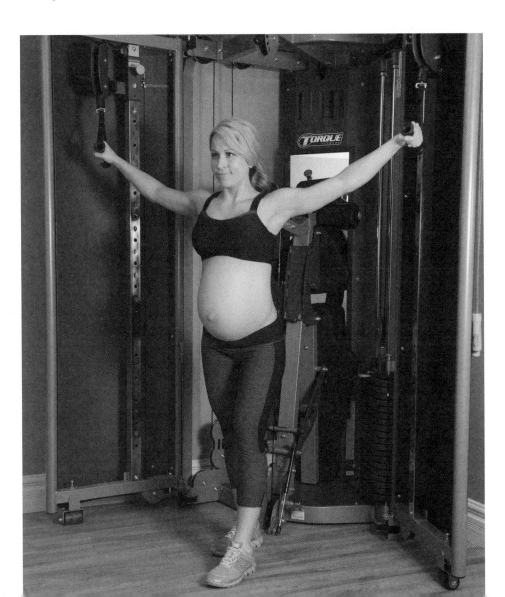

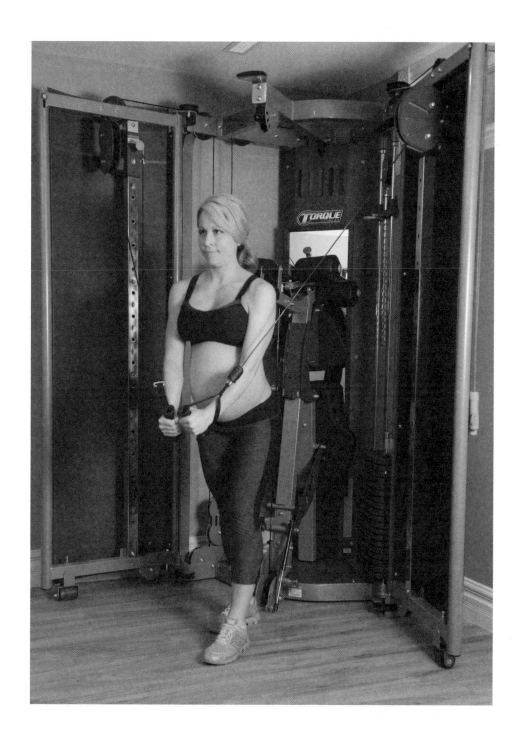

Curtsy Lunges As you progress in your pregnancy, just use your own body weight to perform this move or choose light dumbbells.

1 Stand with your feet shoulder width apart and a dumbbell in each hand.

2 Take a big step back with your left leg, crossing it behind your right. Bend your knees and lower your hips until your right thigh is nearly parallel to the floor. Ensure your front knee doesn't go past your toes.

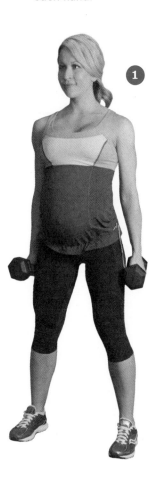

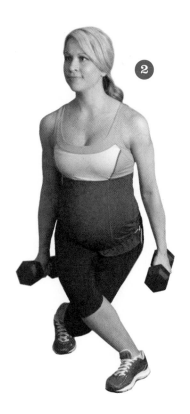

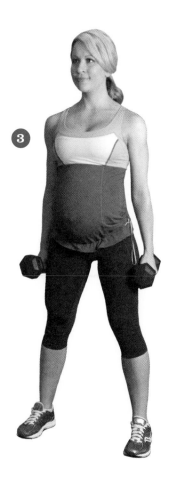

3 Return back to the starting position.

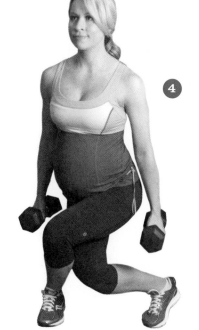

4 Repeat the motion with the other leg to complete 1 repetition.

Deadlift This is an exercise that should be performed only if you are willing to learn how to execute this lift with excellent form and have an experienced trainer review your form. Keep the weight light and focus on form. This lift is included to improve and maintain strength in your low back throughout your pregnancy.

1 Hold the bar with your left palm facing away from you, and your right palm toward you (underhand/overhand grip). Your hands should be placed slightly farther than shoulder width, just outside of your legs. This grip keeps the bar balanced.

2 Feet are inside shoulder width and toes are straight, knees bent.

3 Hips are dropped and back. Mid and low back are dipped in. If at any time you lose this dipping in, stop your set. Your back can lose proper form and round because of fatigue or too much weight.

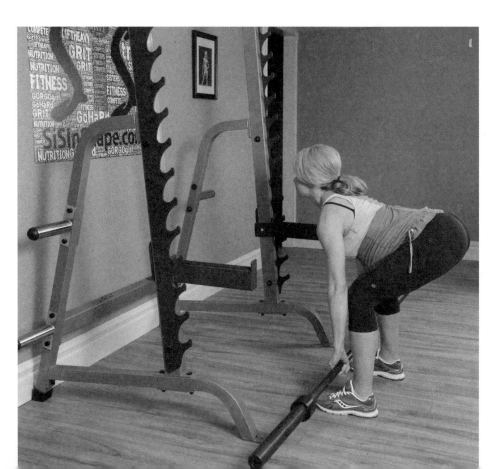

4 Look up at an angle instead of looking straight. When the head tilts back it raises your chest up and keeps you in line.

5 Drag the bar against the shin, over the knee, and up the front of the quad as you stand. Bring it down in the same fashion.

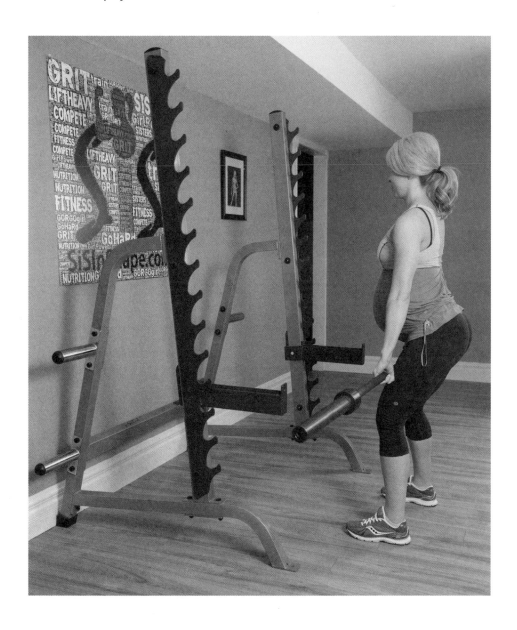

Dumbbell Punches
Give your entire arms a workout with this dynamic move.

1   Hold a light dumbbell in each hand. Feet are slightly farther than shoulder width apart.

2   In a controlled motion, punch your right hand, then your left hand, back and forth slightly above chest height until you've reach the prescribed repetitions.

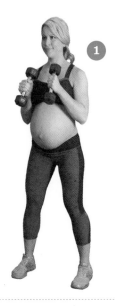

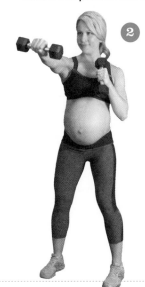

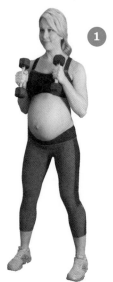

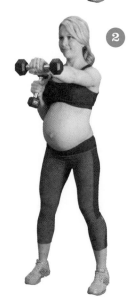

Evil 18s This exercise is performed with three back-to-back shoulder movements of 6 reps for each of the three moves (for a total of 18 reps per set from 6 candlestick front raises + 6 upright rows + 6 overhead presses).

ONE: CANDLESTICK FRONT RAISES

1 Hold a dumbbell in each hand with palms facing each other, thumbs up (like you would hold a candlestick), dumbbells lightly resting on the front of your thighs.

2 Raise the dumbbells up to shoulder height, keeping your palms facing together and arms relatively straight. Come out from your thighs in a V.

3 Lower to your thighs and repeat for a total of 6 reps.

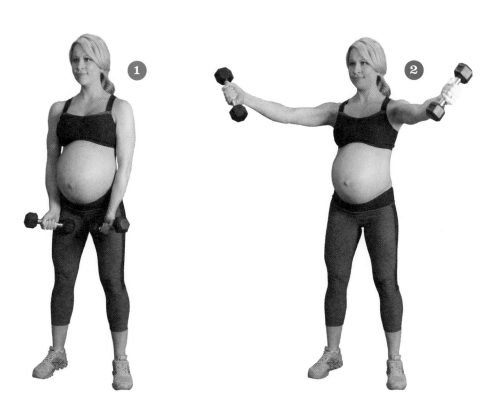

TWO: UPRIGHT ROW WITH DUMBBELLS

1 Hold a dumbbell in each hand with palms facing toward your thighs, dumbbells lightly resting on the front of your thighs.

2 While bending your elbows outward, pull the dumbbells up to chest height.

3 Lower to your thighs and repeat for a total of 6 reps.

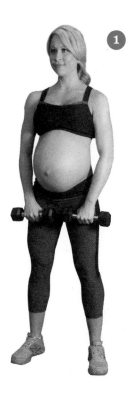

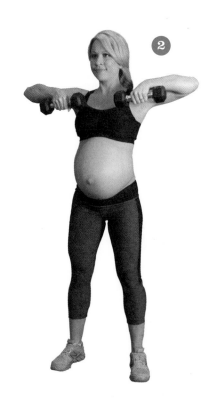

THREE: OVERHEAD DUMBBELL PRESS

1 Flip the dumbbells so both of your palms are facing out and the dumbbells are being held above your shoulders, elbows out.

2 Press the dumbbells overhead so they almost touch.

3 Lower to shoulder height and repeat for a total of 6 reps.

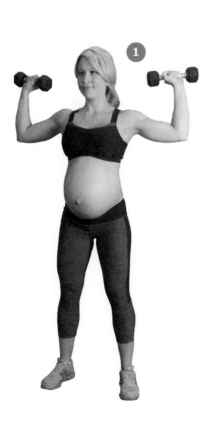

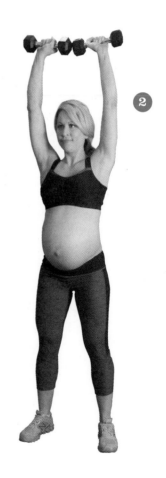

Face Pull with Rope

Attach rope handle to the cable machine in the top position. Stand facing the rope, almost arm's length away from the rope, with your feet shoulder width apart.

1 Grasp the rope and pull the rope toward your face. Keep your low back tucked in and chest high. You should feel this in your upper back (lats) and rear shoulders.

2 Slowly return to the top position and repeat the movement for the prescribed number of repetitions.

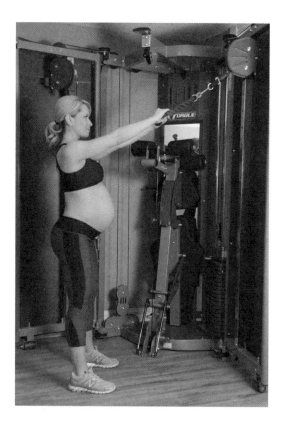
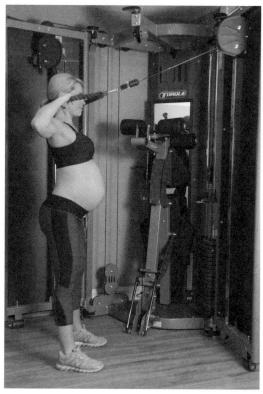

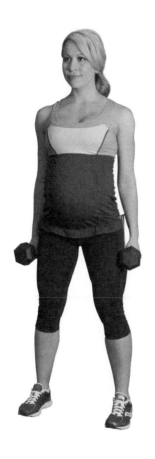

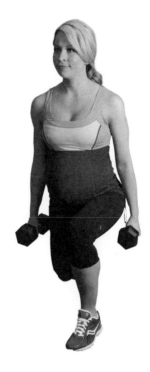

Front Lunge
Stand with a dumbbell in each hand, palms facing toward your thighs. Feet are slightly closer than shoulder width apart.

1 Step forward with your right foot and drop your back knee toward the floor. Your back knee stays a few inches off the floor and your front knee does not go past your right toes.

2 Push your right foot back and focus on pushing your weight through the heel of your front leg.

3 Repeat on the opposite side to complete 1 repetition.

Front Raise with Dumbbells
Stand with feet shoulder width apart and a dumbbell in each hand.

1 Hold the dumbbells against the front of your thighs, palms facing toward your thighs.

2 Raise your right arm in front of you and away from your thighs until it reaches shoulder height.

3 Slowly lower your arm back to your thighs.

4 Switch to your left side to complete 1 repetition.

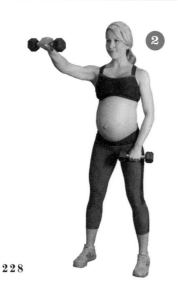

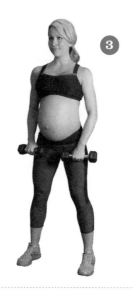

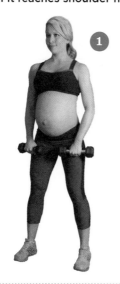

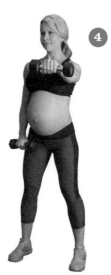

Glute Bridge on BOSU

Sit on the floor a foot away from the BOSU and lean back. Ensure that your back is inclined on the BOSU.

1 Digging your heels into the floor, thrust upward through your hips until your legs form a 90-degree angle with the floor.

2 Hold at the top for 2–3 seconds and squeeze through your glutes.

3 Lower your bum back to the floor to complete 1 repetition.

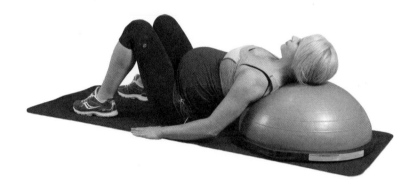

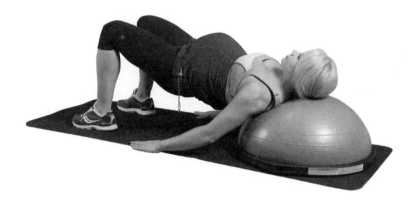

Goblet Sumo Squat   This is an exercise that should be performed only if you are willing to learn how to execute this lift with excellent form and have an experienced trainer review your form. Keep the weight light.

1 Hold a single dumbbell goblet style, as shown. Stand with your feet wide. Toes are pointing to 2 and 10 o'clock.

2 Your low back should be naturally tucked in, and your chest should be high. Look up slightly.

3 Think about keeping your weight on your heels as you squat down. Imagine that you are trying to put your bottom on a little stool that is behind you, as this will help ensure that your knees stay over your feet for knee safety.

4 Only go as low as your balance will safely permit.

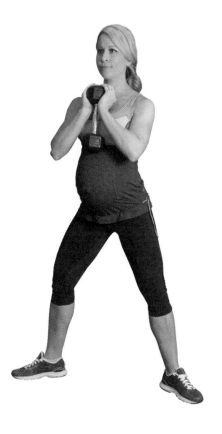
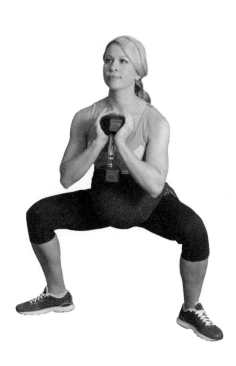

Hammer Curl
Stand or sit at the end of a bench. Your low back should be in, and your chest should be high.

1 Hold the dumbbell as shown so that your thumb is up. Keep your elbows tight. No swinging.

2 Try to touch the dumbbell to your front shoulder.

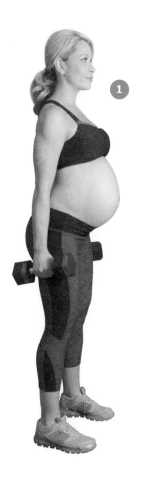

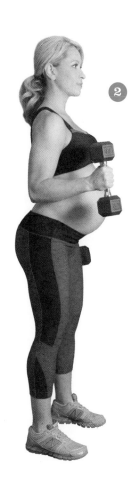

Hands-out Push-up   This push-up variation works your chest and back.

1 From the push-up position (modified on your knees or regular) position your hands so your fingers are pointed outward. Your hands are wider than shoulder width.

2 Keeping your spine in alignment and back straight, lower your chest to the floor (or until your belly just touches the floor) and come back up to full extension.

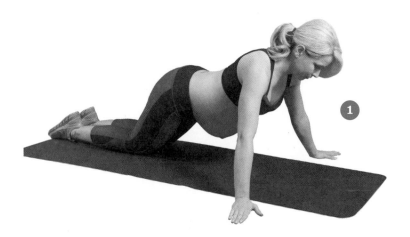

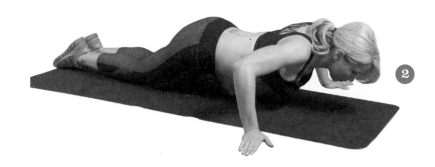

Incline Chest Flye
Position a bench on an incline (about 45 degrees). Sit on the bench with your back against the incline.

1 Dumbbells are positioned straight in front of your chest, palms facing each other and dumbbells touching.

2 Open your arms until your hands are in alignment with your chest.

3 Reverse the movement to complete 1 repetition.

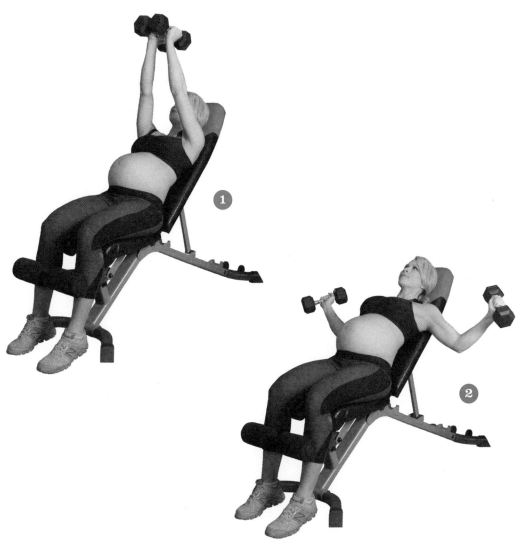

Incline Chest Press
Position a bench on an incline (about 45 degrees). Sit on the bench with your back against the incline.

1 Dumbbells are positioned in front of you, slightly off your chest. Palms are facing outward with the dumbbells held just above your shoulders.

2 Press the dumbbells up and touch them together gently.

3 Reverse the movement to complete 1 repetition.

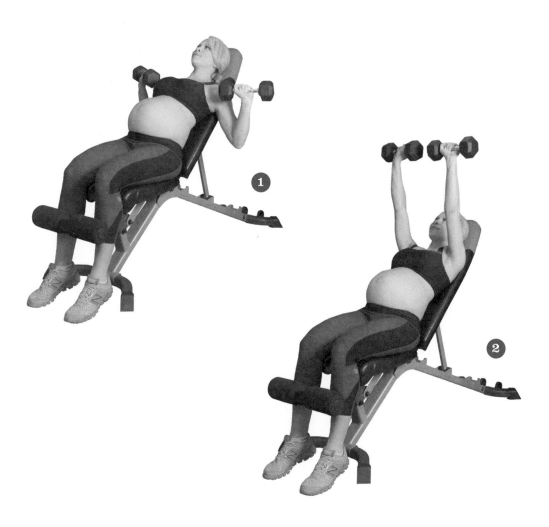

Leaning Side Lateral With a dumbbell in your right hand, held gently against your right thigh, palm facing in, and grab a sturdy object with your left hand (e.g., a cable machine).

1 Keep your feet together and only a few inches away from the object you are holding on to. Lean toward your right until your left arm is straight. Keep your body in alignment.

2 Raise your right arm away from your side until the dumbbell reaches shoulder height. Reverse the movement to complete the repetition.

3 Once all repetitions on one side are complete, switch sides to complete the set.

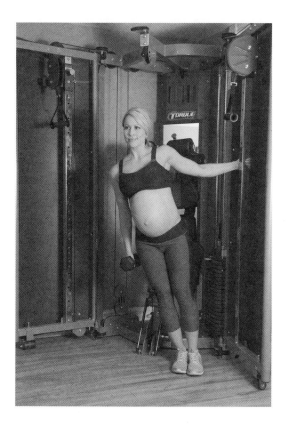

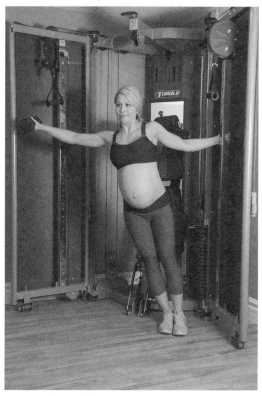

Leg Extension (Toes out) Position yourself on a leg extension machine and adjust the machine to fit your body.

1 Toes are pointed outward.

2 Control the motion as you move your legs up and down. Avoid slinging the weight. Flex slightly in the top position.

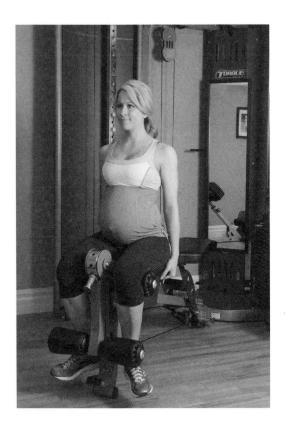

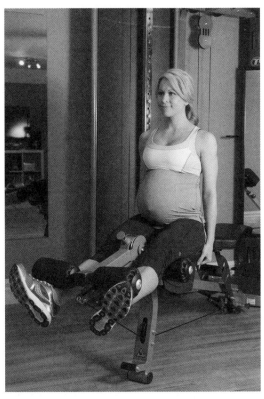

Leg Extension (Toes Straight)
Position yourself in a leg extension machine and adjust the machine to fit your body.

1 Toes are in standard position, pointed straight in front of you.

2 Control the motion as you move your legs up and down. Avoid slinging the weight. Flex slightly in the top position.

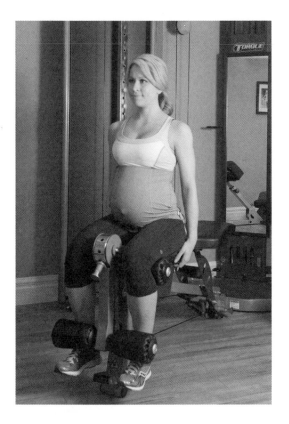
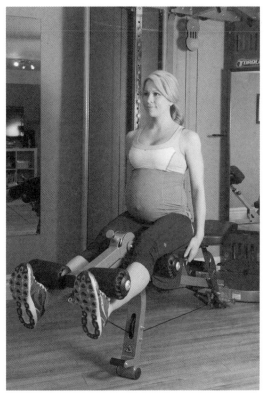

Lunge on BOSU   Use your body weight for this exercise.

1 Face away from the BOSU and extend your right leg backward by placing your right toe on the top of the BOSU.

2 Your front (left) leg is straight.

3 Drop your back (right) knee toward the floor, ensuring your front knee does not go past your toes.

4 Push through your front left heel to straighten back up.

5 Repeat the motion on the same leg for the prescribed number of repetitions before switching sides to complete the set.

Overhead Tricep Extension (One Arm)   Stand with your feet shoulder width apart and a dumbbell in your right hand. Bring your right arm up beside your face, your elbow pointed out and the dumbbell over your head.

1 Using your tricep, extend your arm until it is straight over your head.

2 Reverse the motion to complete 1 repetition, and repeat on the right side for the prescribed number of repetitions.

3 Switch the dumbbell to your left side and follow the same movement for your left tricep to complete the set.

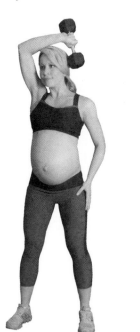
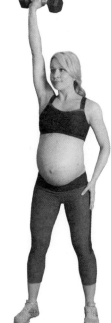

Parallel-grip Lat Pull-down
Attach a triangle bar to the lat pull-down cable machine. Grip the handle so your palms are facing each other. Sit down on the lat pull-down seat. Your low back should be in and your chest should be high.

1 Pull the attachment down to chest level.

2 Using constant tension, reverse the movement to complete 1 repetition.

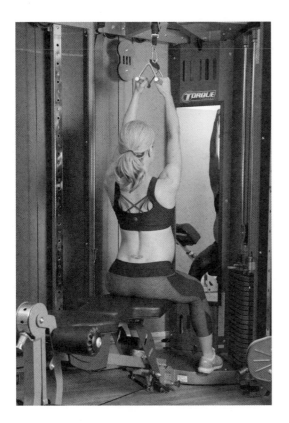
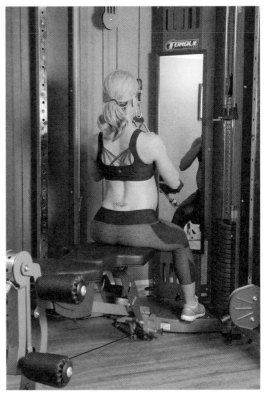

Plate Halo If a plate isn't available, use one dumbbell and grasp it at each end.

1 Firmly grasp a plate with two hands and bring it in front of you at chest height. Arms are straight.

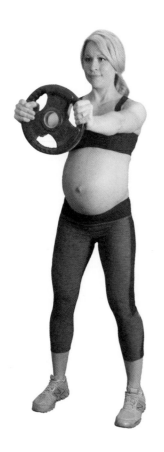

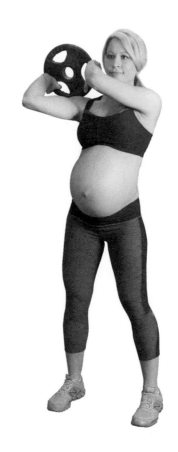

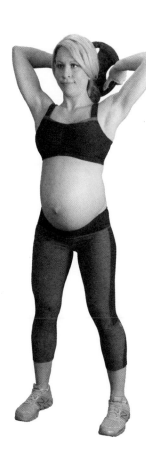

2 Bend your elbows as you move the plate around your head in a clockwise motion until you've returned to the starting position.

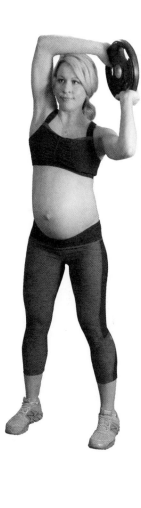

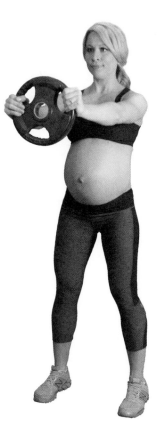

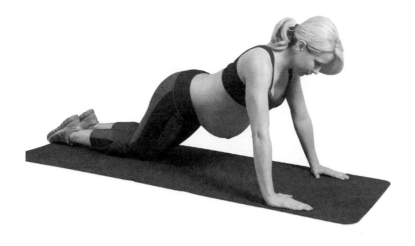

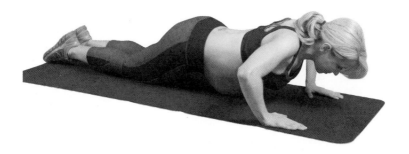

Preggo Push-up

From the push-up position (modified on your knees), position your hands slightly wider than shoulder width apart and fingers pointed forward.

1 Keeping your neck in alignment and back straight, bend your arms and your chest until your belly just touches the floor and come back up to full extension.

Rear Delt Cable Pull

Set the dual cable system to the high setting with the standard handles attached on each pulley. Face the cable machine and hold the handles so that the cables are crisscrossed in front of your face. Feet are shoulder width apart.

1 Start the movement with your wrists crossed and arms slightly bent as if you were hugging a barrel.

2 Pull the cables out wide, keeping a slight bend in your elbows and focusing on pulling with the backs of your shoulders.

3 Slowly reverse the movement to complete 1 repetition.

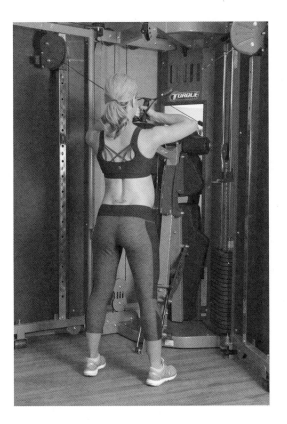 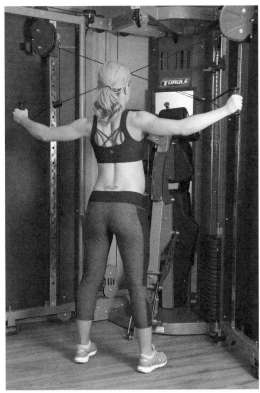

Rear Delt Flye (Standing Wide Legged)
Holding a dumbbell in each hand, palms facing the sides of your legs, stand with your feet wider than shoulder width apart (far enough apart to accommodate your baby belly).

1 Hinging at the hips, bend forward. Ensure that you keep your low back naturally tucked in and chest high. Your neck stays in alignment with your spine.

2 Start with your arms hanging down in front of you and your dumbbells together.

3 Slowly move your arms apart until your arms are in line with your shoulders.

4 Slowly lower the dumbbells to complete 1 repetition.

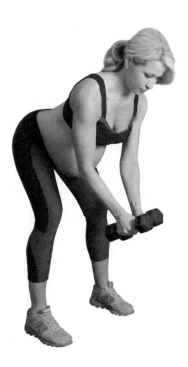
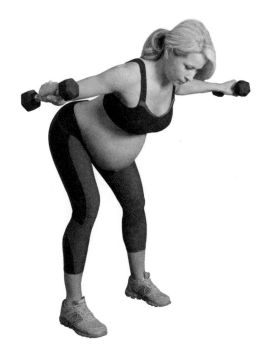

Reverse-grip Lat Pull-down

Sit down on the lat pull-down seat. Grip the overhead handle so that your palms are toward your face. Your hands should be close together. Your low back should be in and your chest should be high.

1 Pull the attachment down to chest level.

2 Using constant tension, reverse the movement to complete 1 repetition.

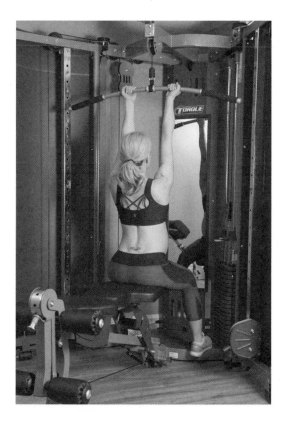
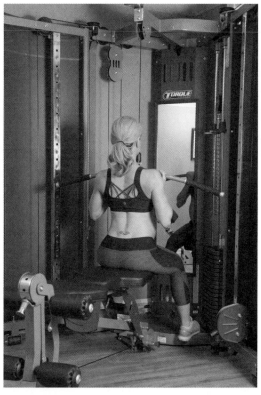

Rope Pull-down
Attach a rope handle to a cable machine in the top position. Stand facing the rope, almost at arm's length away from the rope, with your feet shoulder width apart.

1 Grasp the rope. Keep only a slight bend in your elbows as you pull the rope to your thighs. Keep your low back tucked in and chest high. You should feel this in your upper back (lats).

2 Slowly return to the top position and repeat the movement for the prescribed number of repetitions.

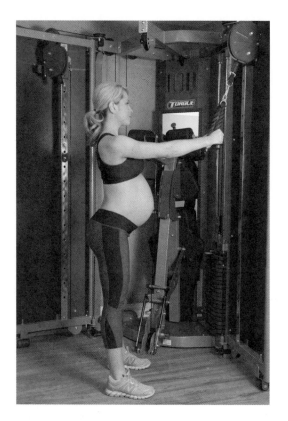

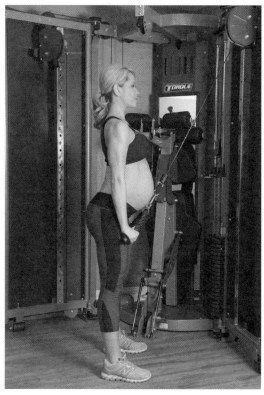

Seated Lateral Raises
Sit on the end of a bench, holding a dumbbell in each hand.

1 Hold the dumbbells against the sides of your thighs, palms facing toward your thighs.

2 Raise both of your arms away from your thighs until they reach shoulder height.

3 Slowly lower your arms back to your thighs to complete the repetition.

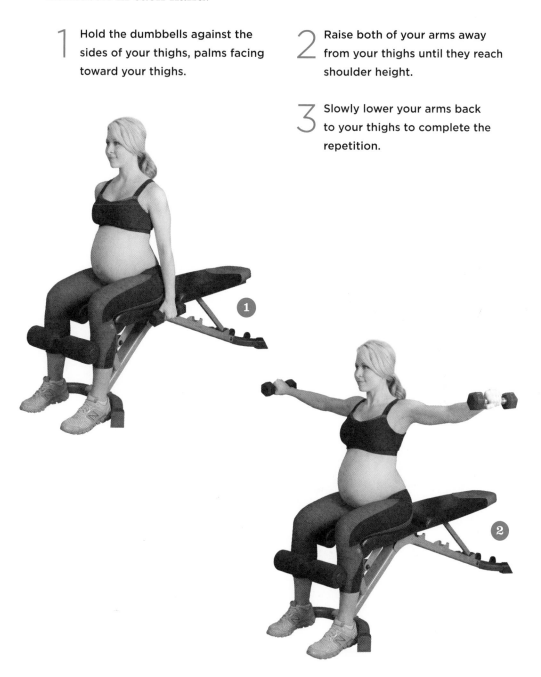

Seated Shoulder Press
Sit on an exercise bench with your back supported. Feet are flat on the floor.

1 Hold a dumbbell in each hand at shoulder height. Elbows are bent at 90 degrees and your palms are facing away from you.

2 Press your hands overhead until the dumbbells touch.

3 Reverse the motion to complete 1 repetition.

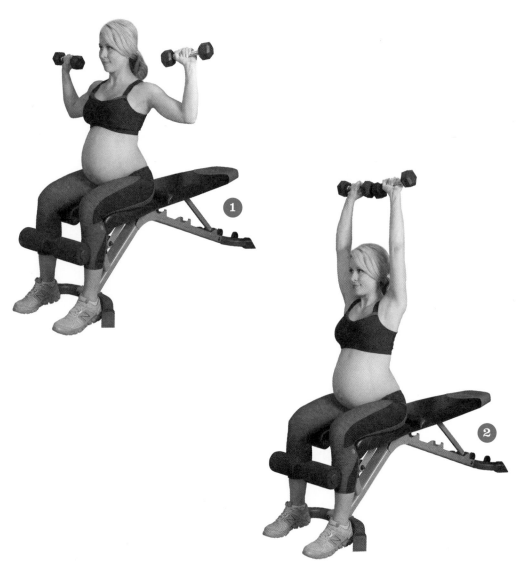

Side Lateral Raise
Stand with feet shoulder width apart and a dumbbell in each hand.

1 Hold the dumbbells against the sides of your thighs, palms facing toward your thighs.

2 Raise both of your arms away from your thighs until they reach shoulder height.

3 Slowly lower your arms back to your thighs to complete the repetition.

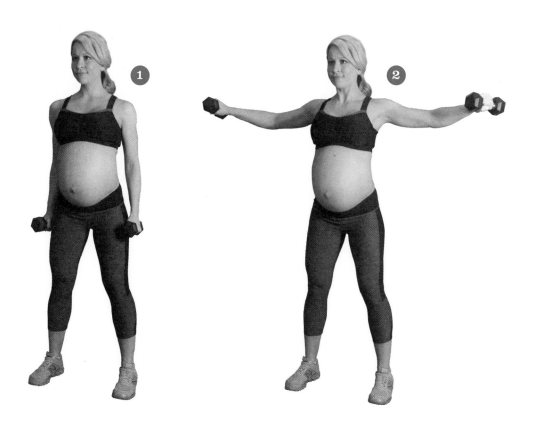

Side Plank
Lie on your right side with your right arm underneath you at a 90-degree angle from your body and your feet stacked on top of each other.

1 Using your bent right arm for stabilization, bring your hips off the mat so that your body is in alignment.

2 Hold the side plank for the prescribed time. Stop if you feel your core weaken or your midline give out.

3 Switch to your left side and repeat the motions on your left side to complete 1 set.

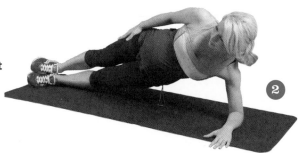

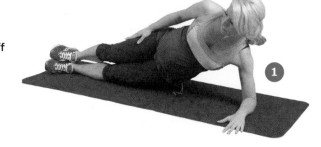

Side Squat on BOSU
Use your body weight for this exercise.

1 Stand beside a BOSU and place your right foot on the top of the BOSU. Your left leg is straight. Your low back should naturally tucked in and your chest should be high.

2 Think about keeping your weight on your left heel as you squat down. Imagine that you are trying to put your bottom on a little stool that is behind you as this

will help ensure that your knees stay over your feet for knee safety.

3 Push back up through the weight in your left heel.

4 Repeat the motion on the same leg for the prescribed number of repetitions before switching sides to complete the set.

Single-Arm Row on Bench

Place a dumbbell on each side of a flat bench. Put your left knee on top of the end of the bench, and your left hand on the other end of the bench for support.

1 Use your right hand to pick up the dumbbell on the floor, palm facing toward the bench. Throughout the entire movement keep your low back naturally tucked in and chest high. Your neck stays in alignment with your spine.

2 Pull the dumbbell straight up to the side of your chest, keeping your arm close to your side.

3 Lower the weight to complete 1 repetition. Complete all repetitions on one side before switching to the other side.

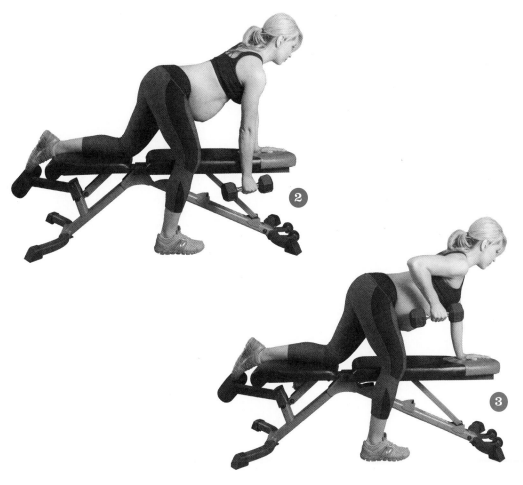

Squat This is an exercise that should be performed only if you are willing to learn how to execute this lift with excellent form and have an experienced trainer review your form. Keep the weight light or use only your body weight. If you are using a barbell, the use of a squat rack is encouraged so you are not hoisting the weight over your head. You can hold a dumbbell in each hand to avoid lifting the weight overhead.

1 Stand with your feet slightly apart, slightly more than shoulder width. Toes are pointing to 1 and 11 o'clock.

2 Your low back should be naturally tucked in and your chest should be high. Look up.

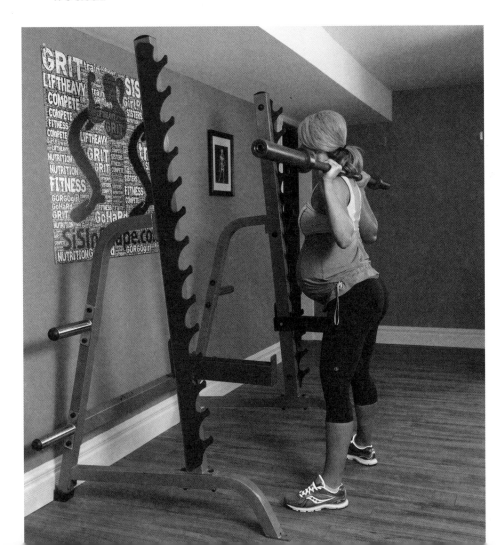

3 Think about keeping your weight on your heels as you squat down. Imagine that you are trying to put your bottom on a little stool that is behind you as this will help ensure that your knees stay over your feet for knee safety.

4 Only squat down as low as you feel you can do safely. Ideally, the goal is be able to break parallel with the depth of your squat.

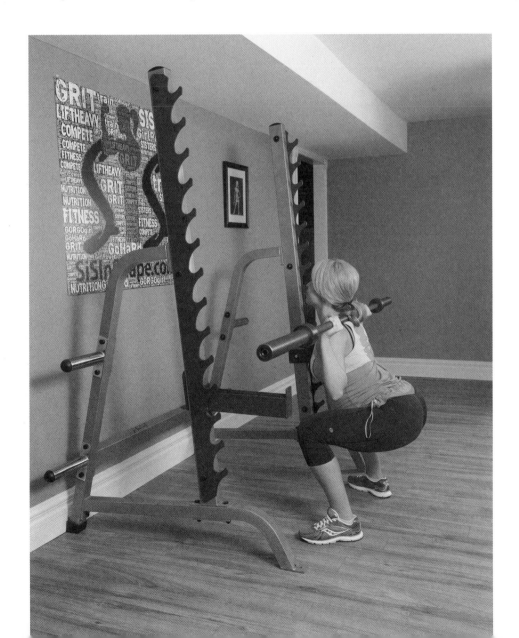

Standing Kickback on Cable Machine

Attach a standard handle and adjust the cable pulley to the bottom position. Face the cable machine and hold on to the machine for balance.

1 With feet shoulder width apart, hook the toes of your right foot into the standard handle.

2 Keeping your spine in alignment and holding the machine for balance, take the right leg back and diagonal.

3 Squeeze your glute and slowly return to starting position.

4 Repeat for the prescribed number of repetitions.

5 Once the right side repetitions are complete, switch sides to finish the set.

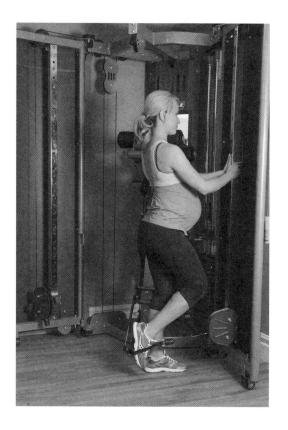
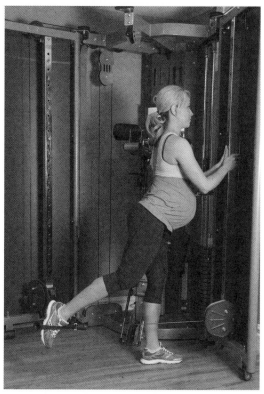

Tricep Rope Extension
Secure the rope attachment to the cable pulley machine. Stand in front of the rope attachment with your feet shoulder width apart.

1 Grasp the rope with each hand and lower the rope so it is slightly below chest height.

2 Press the rope down until your arms are fully extended and your hands are close to your thighs.

3 Using constant tension, reverse the motion to slightly below chest height to complete 1 repetition.

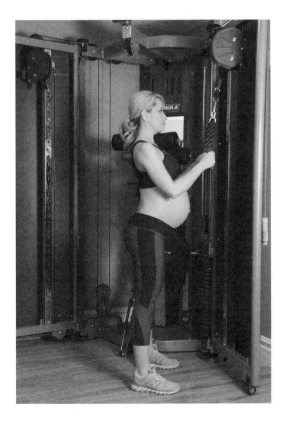
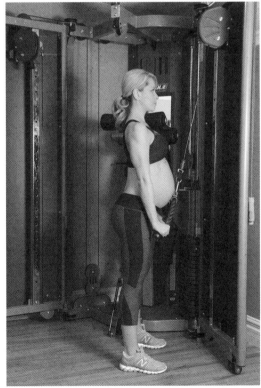

Step-ups on Bench
Go slow and choose a light weight (or no weight). If you have any concerns about your balance, swap this move for a front lunge.

1 Stand in front of a flat bench or exercise step. Place your left foot in the middle, on top of the bench.

2 Shift your weight into your left heel as you step up onto the bench. The focus here is on your left leg so your right foot comes up onto the bench only to be tapped on the bench or to balance yourself before you place your right foot back on the floor.

3 Keep your left foot on the bench and repeat the motion for the prescribed number of repetitions.

4 Switch to the right leg and follow the same movement for the prescribed number of repetitions to complete the set.

Tricep Dip on Bench
Position yourself about a foot away from a flat bench. The bench is behind you.

1 Grip the edge of the bench with your hands behind you so that your wrists are facing your back. Your hands are shoulder width apart. Your legs are extended forward with a slight bend in the knee.

2 Slowly lower your body by bending at the elbows until your arms are bent at 90 degrees.

3 Press up through your triceps to complete the motion.

4 Repeat the lower and press-up motion for the prescribed number of repetitions.

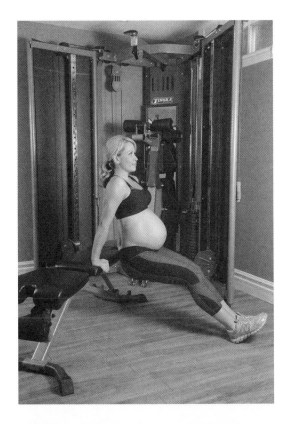

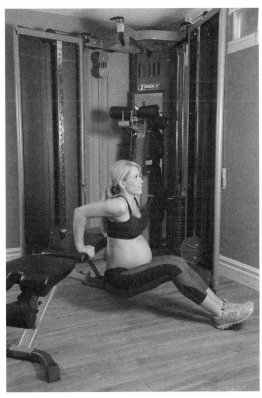

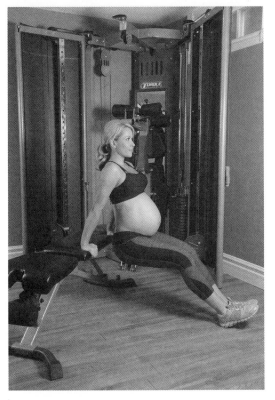

Upright Chest Press

Perform this exercise on a seated chest press machine, or stand in between two cable pulleys, attach two standard handles to the cable machine, and set the height to your chest height.

1 Grasp each handle and bring your hands in line with your shoulders. Elbows are bent.

of you. Ensure that you keep your core tight and your spine in a neutral position.

2 Press your hands forward until your arms are straight out in front

3 Return to the starting position to complete 1 repetition.

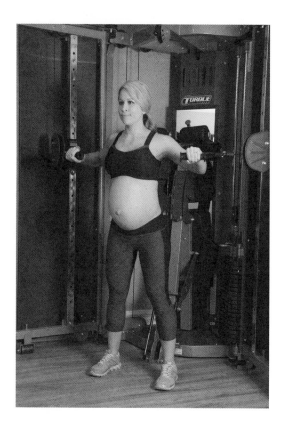
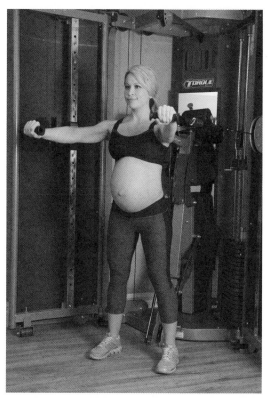

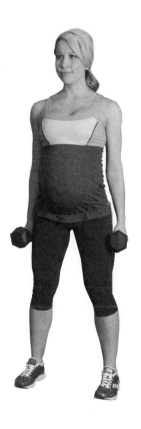
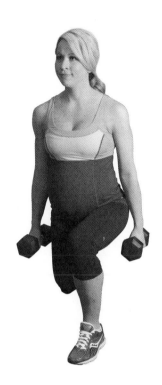
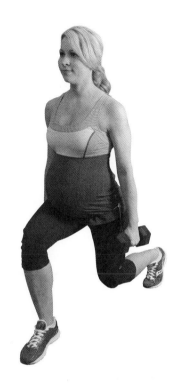

Walking Lunges
Stand with a dumbbell in each hand, palms facing toward your thighs. Feet are slightly closer than shoulder width.

1 Step forward with your right foot and drop your back knee toward the floor. Your back knee stays a few inches off the floor.

2 With the weight in your front right heel, bring your left leg forward and step in front of your right leg.

3 Drop your right (back) knee toward the floor, keeping it a few inches off the floor.

4 With the weight in your front left heel, bring your right leg forward and step in front of your left leg. That is 1 repetition.

5 Continue "walking" in this manner for the prescribed number of repetitions.

Wall Sit Stand against a wall and slowly lower yourself into a seated position. Your feet should be far enough away to ensure that your knees do not go past your toes.

1 Hold the "sit" while focusing on the strength it takes in your thighs and glutes.

2 If you feel pressure in your pelvic floor, stop the exercise.

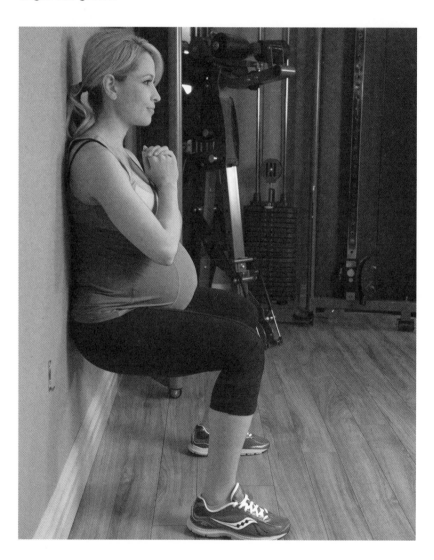

Wide-grip Lat Pull-down

Sit down on the lat pull-down seat. Grip the overhead handle so that your palms are away from your face and your hands are wider than shoulder width. Your low back should be in, and your chest should be high.

1 Pull the attachment down to chest level.

2 Using constant tension, reverse the movement to complete 1 repetition.

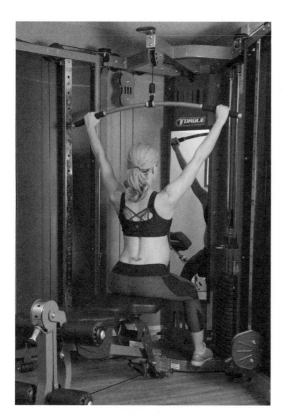
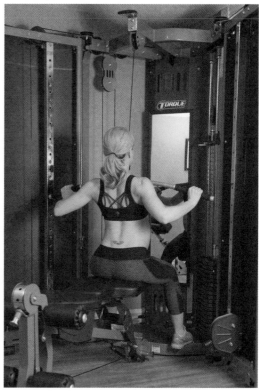

Model: Andrea Bradley (my sister!)

Cat-Cow During pregnancy, Cat pose and Cow pose are both great for low back pain. They give a gentle stretch for both the low back and abdominal muscles.

1 Starting on your hands and knees, ensure that your wrists and hands are aligned underneath your shoulders and that your knees are positioned below your hips.

2 Your feet are flexed, soles up, with your legs a little more than hip width apart to make space for your belly.

3 Your palms should be flat on the mat and fingers facing forward.

4 Inhale, stretch your neck, and lift your head forward and chest up. Lift your tailbone and drop your belly toward the ground.

5 Exhale, drop your belly in and up, curl your spine out, and roll your tailbone and chin toward each other.

6 Repeat for 8–15 breaths.

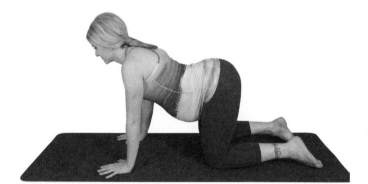

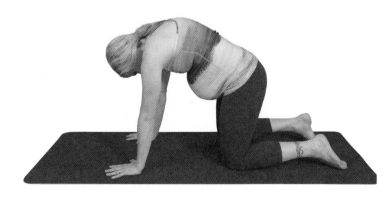

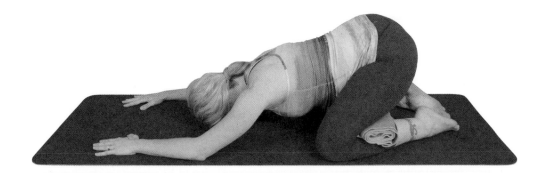

Child Pose This is a restorative pose that stretches your hips and also gives your low back a gentle stretch.

1 Starting on your hands and knees, ensure that your wrists and hands are aligned underneath your shoulders and that your knees are positioned below your hips.

2 Your feet are placed along the mat, soles up, with your legs a little more than hip width apart to make space for your belly as you drop your hips down to your heels.

3 Use a towel behind your knees if you cannot get your hips all the way down toward your heels.

4 Drop your chest toward the floor so your arms are straight ahead on the mat and your head is resting on the ground. Another option is to put your hands into fists and rest your head on your fists instead of the mat.

5 Breathe for 10–20 breaths.

L-Standing Supported by Wall
This pose strengthens your core and chest muscles. It also gives the back of your legs—your hamstrings—a gentle stretch.

1 Stand in front of a wall at arm's length, feet a bit more than shoulder width apart to make room for your belly. Reach forward from your shoulders and put your palms on the wall, fingers wide and pointing at the ceiling.

2 Keeping your spine neutral (do not arch), begin to walk your legs back, folding at the waist, and walking your hands down the wall. Eventually you'll come to an L shape, as shown in the photo.

3 Don't strain to go farther. You're looking for a nice gentle stretch, not a forward crunch.

4 Slowly inhale and exhale for 10–20 breaths before moving on to the next pose.

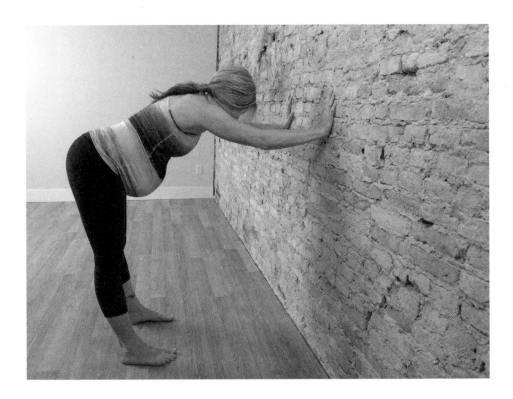

Partner Heart and Butterfly

This is a comforting stretch that you can do you with a partner. It offers a gentle stretch for the front of your body and a relaxing pose you can do with baby's daddy or a friend.

1   Start with mom and her partner in Butterfly with their backs against each other. For Butterfly, bend the knees and bring the soles of the feet together with knees open toward the mat.

2   On an exhale, her partner will begin to fold forward, while mom inhales into a gentle backbend.

3   Hold here for a few breaths, and then her partner inhales, lifting up, taking mom and her partner back to the starting position.

4   Mom then exhales into the fold, taking her partner into a backbend.

5   Repeat this sequence for 8–10 breaths.

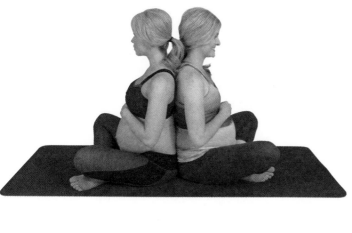

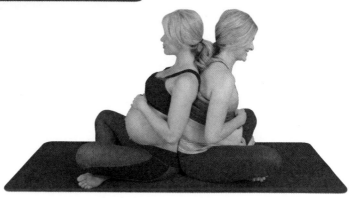

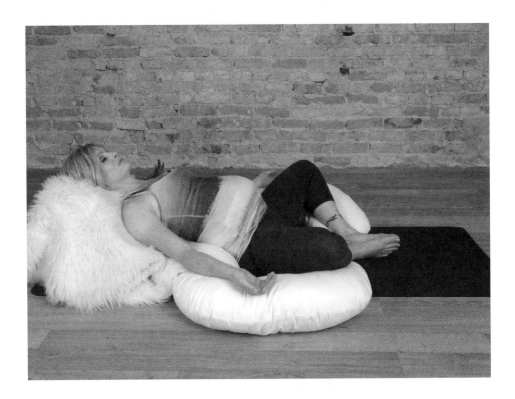

Reclining Butterfly Supported with Pillows

This pose gently opens your hips as you connect with baby.

1 Place 1-2 bolsters or pillows on your mat. If you have a sensitive back, you can create an angle with the bolster by placing a block underneath.

2 Sit with your pelvis close to the edge of the bolster and lie so that the bolster raises the pelvis.

3 Choose a comfortable position for the legs, either bent or with the knees apart in Butterfly. For Butterfly, bend the knees and bring the soles of the feet together with knees open toward the mat.

4 Stay in this pose for 2–4 minutes, breathing in and out with the intention of connecting with your baby.

Runner's Lunge with Block
This pose stretches and strengthens your quadriceps and hamstrings. It also helps strengthen your core muscles.

1 With a block placed on your right, stand with feet slightly wider than shoulder width to give you room for your belly.

2 Step back with your right foot and slowly come down to your right knee, using the block on your right side for stability. Lay the top of your right foot along the mat and rest your left arm just above your bent left knee.

3 Make sure your left knee does not extend forward but is stacked above your ankle, and press down slightly with your right hip toward the floor.

4 Breathe slowly for 10–20 breaths, then switch sides to repeat.

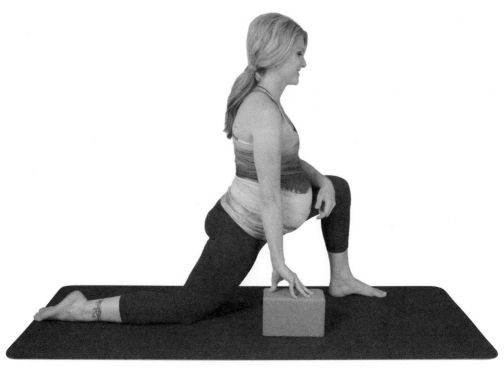

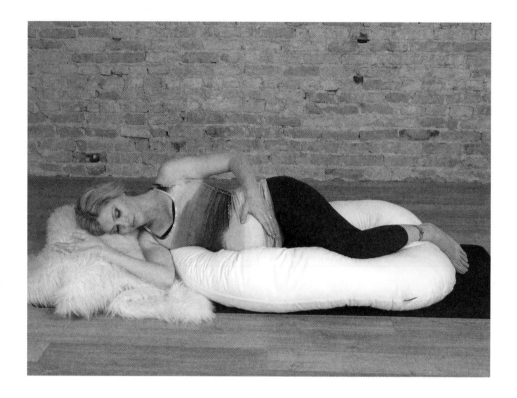

Side-lying Pose Supported with Pillows

This restorative pose allows you to connect with baby while calming your nervous system.

1 Lie on your side with your top knee bent and supported by a pillow. You can also place a long pillow or stacked blankets under your belly and your head.

2 Place a pillow in between your legs to help keep your hips in alignment.

3 Place your hand on your belly and close your eyes. Focus on your breath. With each breath, connect with yourself and baby.

Seated Wide-Legged Straddle with Chest Twist

This pose stretches the hamstrings and calves, and elongates the spine.

1 From a seated position on the floor, open the legs out as wide as comfortable. If you need to, prop a rolled towel under your sit bones.

2 Keep the thigh muscles engaged and feet flexed, toes pointing up.

3 Press the legs down into the floor.

4 For stability, put your left hand in between your legs and right hand slightly behind you. Gently twist from your chest, not your abdomen, toward the right for a nice gentle stretch. Keep your hips and abdomen forward. Do not force the twist. Breathe 10–20 times.

5 Switch hands and repeat on the other side.

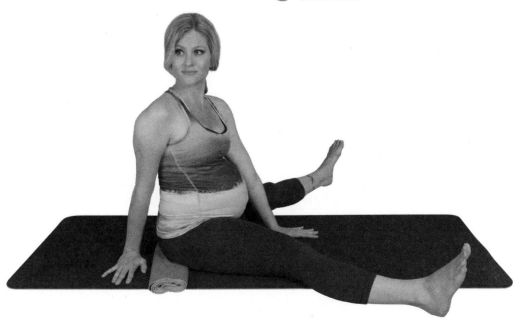

Spinal Balance Pose

This pose strengthens your core and low back.

1 Starting on your hands and knees, ensure your wrists and hands are aligned underneath your shoulders and that your knees are positioned below your hips.

2 Your feet are flexed, soles up, with your legs a little more than hip width apart to make space for your belly.

3 Keep your eyes looking at the mat to keep your spine in alignment. Your spine should be kept neutral throughout the pose.

4 Inhale as you reach your right arm forward until it is straight out in front of you next to your ear. Raise your left leg off the mat, ensuring that you do not raise your leg past your hips. Hold for a count of two.

5 Exhale and return to the starting position. Repeat on the opposite side for 5–10 repetitions on each side.

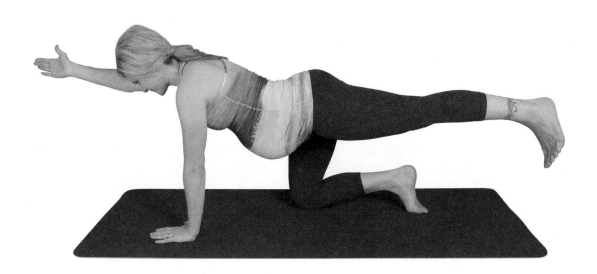

Standing Quad Stretch Supported by Wall
This pose stretches the front of your legs and chest while helping you develop balance.

1 Stand with your left side next to the wall, and place your left hand on the wall for stability.

2 Bend your right knee, bring your right foot up to your bottom, and hold your right foot with your right hand.

3 Keep your right knee in alignment with your hips and gently stretch the front of your quad. Your spine should stay neutral (do not arch).

4 Breathe for 10–20 breaths before switching to the other side to repeat the motion.

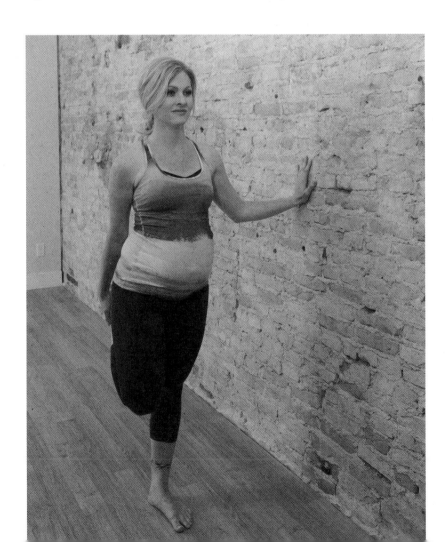

Notes

Chapter 1

p. 7: *It is a well-accepted guideline . . .* Mayo Clinic Staff, "Pregnancy Weight Gain: What's Healthy?" Mayo Clinic website, http://www.mayoclinic.org/ healthy-living/ pregnancy-week-by-week/ in-depth/pregnancy-weight-gain/art-20044360.

p. 8: *The Spartans believed . . .* Stephanie Lynn Budin, *The Ancient Greeks: New Perspectives* (Santa Barbara, CA: ABC-CLIO, 2004), p. 145.

p. 9: *Mommy and Baby Benefits of Exercising during Pregnancy* Mayo Clinic Staff, "Pregnancy and Exercise: Baby, Let's Move!" Mayo Clinic website, http:// www.mayoclinic.org/healthy-living/ pregnancy-week-by-week/in-depth/ pregnancy-and-exercise/art-20046896.

p. 9: *Boosts baby's brain maturity* "Mom's Exercise during Pregnancy Gives Baby's Brain a Boost," CBC News, November 11, 2013, http://www.cbc.ca/ news/health/mom-s-exercise-during-pregnancy-gives-baby-s-brain-a-boost-1.2422831.

p. 9: *Lowers gestational diabetes risk* C. Zhang, "Adherence to Healthy Lifestyle and Risk of Gestational Diabetes Mellitus: Prospective Cohort Study," *BMJ*, September 30, 2014, http:// www.bmj.com/content/349/bmj.g5450; Roxanne Nelson, "Pre-pregnancy

Lifestyle Impacts Gestational Diabetes," *Chicago Tribune*, October 14, 2014, http://www.chicagotribune.com/lifestyles/ health/sns-rt-us-health-pregnancy-diabetes-20141014-story.html.

p. 9: *May boost child's athletic potential . . . lasts into childhood* M. Bahls et al. "Mothers' Exercise during Pregnancy Programs Vasomotor Function in Adult Offspring," *Experimental Physiology* 99, no. 1 (2013): 205–219; Christopher Bergland, "Physical Activity during Pregnancy Benefits Babies' Health," *Psychology Today*, October 2014, https:// www.psychologytoday.com/blog/the-athletes-way/201310/physical-activity-during-pregnancy-benefits-babies-health.

p. 12: *If you deliver vaginally . . .* Se Jin Song, Maria Gloria Dominguez-Bello, and Rob Knight, "How Delivery Mode and Feeding Can Shape the Bacterial Community in the Infant Gut," *Canadian Medical Association Journal* 185, no. 5 (2013): 373–374, http://www.ncbi.nlm. nih.gov/pmc/articles/PMC3602250/.

p. 13: *The nutrients are then absorbed . . .* "Inside Pregnancy: How Food Reaches Your Baby," Baby Centre website, http:// www.babycentre.co.uk/v1049111/inside-pregnancy-how-food-reaches-your-baby-video.

Chapter 2

p. 22: *The AOCG says* . . . Committee on Obstetric Practice, "Exercise during Pregnancy and the Postpartum Period," ACOG Committee Opinion 267. American College of Obstetricians and Gynecologists. *Obstet. Gynecol*. 99 (2002): 171–173, http://www.acog.org/Resources-And-Publications/Committee-Opinions/Committee-on-Obstetric-Practice/Exercise-During-Pregnancy-and-the-Postpartum-Period.

p. 24: *As your heart rate increases* . . . Jenny Hope, "Fit Mothers Have Healthier Babies as Exercise during Pregnancy Strengthens Blood Vessels of Unborn Children," Daily Mail, October 24, 2013. http://www.dailymail.co.uk/health/article-2476292/Fit-mothers-healthier-babies-exercise-pregnancy-strengthens-blood-vessels-unborn-children.html; L. E. May et al., "Regular Maternal Exercise Dose and Fetal Heart Outcome," *Med. Sci. Sports Exerc*. 44, no. 7 (2012): 1252–1258, http://www.ncbi.nlm.nih.gov/pubmed/22217566.

p. 33: *Soy is a controversial topic*. Joseph Mercola, "The Health Dangers of Soy," Huffington Post, August 23, 2012, http://www.huffingtonpost.com/dr-mercola/soy-health_b_1822466.html.

p. 40: *Supplements, including protein powders* . . . "Dietary Supplements," U.S. Food and Drug Administration website, http://www.fda.gov/Food/DietarySupplements/.

Chapter 6

p. 133: *You need 400–500 additional calories* . . . Mayo Clinic Staff, "Breast-Feeding Nutrition: Tips for Moms," Mayo Clinic website, http://www.mayoclinic.org/healthy-living/infant-and-toddler-health/in-depth/breastfeeding-nutrition/art-20046912.

Acknowledgments

LIKE YOUR NEW BABY, this book was not created and delivered alone. There were many special people who breathed life into this book well after I held beautiful baby Faith in my arms.

First is the support of time and encouragement that I received from my mother-in-law Bev. She cared for our kids and household as I researched, interviewed, wrote, and edited this book so that many women could give themselves and their babies the healthiest and fittest start to a new life together. We truly are a family of strength and love.

Dear reader (and girlfriend on this journey), I am incredibly grateful to the experts that allowed me to share their amazing knowledge and gifts with you:

Registered Holistic Nutritionist Christal Sczebel dished her yummy preggo-power recipes among her beautiful food photography. The talents of this one woman are amazing.

The forward-thinking Bellies Inc. team of Kim Vopni, Sam Montpetit-Huynh, and Julia Di Paolo are on a mission to get us women talking about our pelvic floor health. I'll never forget their encouragement of me nursing a fussy baby Faith during our "professional" video interview.

For photographer Carston Leishman of Lemontree Photography to capture so many stunning images of a woman with a huge baby bump in a sports bra, you know he must have an incredible talent.

This book would not have materialized without my book agent Coleen O'Shea and Sterling Publishing editor Kate Zimmerman. These two set this fitness blogger on course to help me navigate the world of publishing and gave me the opportunity to become a true author. Thank you for what you two do.

How amazing are my (your!) Preggo Pals? Meaghan, Katy, Dani, Christie, and Val. The openness of these women to share their stories is a gift and inspiration.

A special note of gratitude to my dear friend Lindsay. By sharing her darkest moments post-partum, and never (ever) giving up, she turned a dark experience into light and hope for many others.

Finally, but not least, is my husband Tim. Thank you for teaching me true love, Tim. While the gifts of love and life have been many from you, it's the gift of true love that I can now pour into our babies and the work that I do that I'm most thankful for. I am forever yours and you know none of this could be accomplished without our togetherness.

About the Author

ERICA WILLICK is a two-time North American fitness competition champion. She earned these titles competing in 2012 and 2013, *after* the birth of her first child in 2010 and while working full-time in a corporate finance job. Erica has appeared in print magazines such as *Oxygen* as both a model and an author. She is also the founder of SISTERS IN SHAPE, an online community where over 15,000 women regularly read Erica's writings and watch her videos on nutrition, fitness, and how to balance it all in real life. Erica is a regular guest on Canada's largest talk radio station, AM 590, as a health and fitness expert, and she also appears as a featured speaker at health and fitness workshops. She is a spokesperson for UFE (Ultimate Fitness Events). Erica is also the CEO of *GORGO Women's Fitness* magazine, which debuted in 2013 and now has over 25,000 subscribers. Her blog—about pre- and postnatal fitness and health—receives about 11,000 hits per weekly post. You can find out more about Erica at sisinshape.com. She lives in Ontario, Canada.

Index